*Francis J. Turner, DSW*

# Diagnosis in Social Work
## *New Imperatives*

*Pre-publication*
REVIEWS,
COMMENTARIES,
EVALUATIONS . . .

"**I**n this book, Francis Turner returns, so to speak, to his roots. Long identified with the 'diagnostic school,' Turner presents a strong defense of this important aspect of professional practice. The text covers a wide range of topics including a history of diagnosis in social work, Turner's views on how this part of practice was subverted, and a consideration of contemporary issues such as the role of computers and technology in diagnosis. For those of use who 'grew up' in social work education and practice in the 1970s and beyond, the chapter contrasting diagnosis and assessment will be most illuminating.

This is an excellent book by a seminal writer who has 'stayed the course' with his convictions and beliefs about what is important in social work practice. For direct practitioners and teachers of direct/micro practice, this is 'must' reading."

**Kenneth I. Millar, PhD**
Dean, School of Social Work,
Louisiana State University,
Baton Rouge

"**I**n his newest book, *Diagnosis in Social Work,* Professor Francis Turner has reviewed the profession's history with a focus on how social workers make decisions about clients and how these decisions are communicated. This review makes clear the reasons for social work's most recent ambivalence about diagnostic work. Professor Turner also makes clear the profession's strengths in assessment and clinical approach and argues the need for diagnosis to solidify social work's role in helping people change their lives. This book is a useful resource for scholars and clinicians involved in clinical social work. It is thoughtfully written, well researched, and a timely addition to the professional literature."

**Kathleen J. Farkas, PhD**
Associate Professor,
Mandel School of Applied
Social Sciences,
Case Western Reserve University,
Cleveland, Ohio

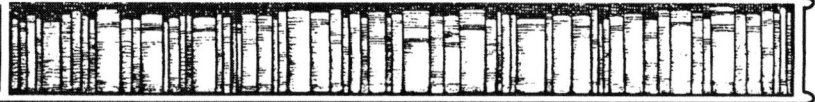

*More pre-publication*
*REVIEWS, COMMENTARIES, EVALUATIONS . . .*

"Turner advocates the importance of precision in communicating client needs when providing service. He suggests that the move from diagnosis to assessment has diluted the clarity with which it is necessary to plan appropriately for and with clients. Turner believes that if we are not more precise in clearly diagnosing conditions, for example, attention-deficit disorder, phobias, or eating disorders, we potentially impede the client's access to service. He further believes that in current health care schemes we disadvantage our clients by not insisting on a social work diagnosis rather than yielding to a type of diagnosis by code that requires restricted categorization and results in limited service.

Turner makes an excellent case for revisiting the implications of using a social work diagnosis. Although the use of assessment was and is an effort to be more inclusive of the client's experience, the changed circumstances of providing social work services should impel us to examine anything that may provide better services to clients. In his book, Dr. Turner offers a new look at the meaning of diagnosis."

**Florence W. Vigilante, DSW**
Editor, *Journal of Teaching in Social Work;*
Professor, Hunter College
School of Social Work,
New York City

"In this wonderful must-read book, Francis Turner challenges social work to reintegrate its unique professional perspective on diagnosis into the practice repertoire of the profession. The book effectively captures the historical role that sound clinical judgment has played in social work, and through Turner's experience-based analysis leads the reader to a contemporary understanding of the importance of diagnosis in practice. This book builds on Turner's commitment to a multitheoretical approach to direct service, and serves as an excellent compendium text to those struck by the limitations of the DSM and the remedicalization of the helping process."

**G. Brent Angell, PhD, LCSW**
Associate Professor
and MSW Program Chair,
School of Social Work
and Criminal Justice Studies,
East Carolina University,
Greenville, North Carolina

"Francis Turner has made another valuable contribution to the social work literature. In *Diagnosis in Social Work: New Imperatives,* he examines the history and changing meaning of the concept of diagnosis in direct practice in social work.

Turner makes a passionate case for the profession to embrace the term diagnosis as the accurate and therefore correct name for what practitioners do within the worker-client helping relationship. He meets the traditional arguments against the use of the term diagnosis by stating what it does not mean and then what it does mean.

Turner's 'diagnosis' is a richly textured, multidimensional, and inevitable process. It is the essence of social work practice. Turner has placed himself with the giants of social work theory: Mary Richmond, Charlotte Towle, Florence Hollis, Gordon Hamilton, and Helen Harris Perlman."

**Luke Fusco, MA**
Dean, Faculty of Social Work,
Wilfrid Laurier University,
Waterloo, Ontario, Canada

# Diagnosis in Social Work
## *New Imperatives*

# Diagnosis in Social Work
## *New Imperatives*

Francis J. Turner, DSW

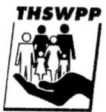

The Haworth Social Work Practice Press
An Imprint of The Haworth Press, Inc.
New York • London • Oxford

Published by

The Haworth Social Work Practice Press, an imprint of The Haworth Press, Inc., 10 Alice Street, Binghamton, NY 13904–1580.

Cases 1, 2, and 3 in the Appendix are from *Social Work Practice: A Canadian Perspective,* F. Turner (Ed.), 1999, pp. 129-130, Toronto: Allyn and Bacon. Reprinted with permission by Pearson Education Canada Inc.

Cover design by Jennifer Gaska.

**Library of Congress Cataloging-in-Publication Data**

Turner, Francis J. (Francis Joseph)
  Diagnosis in social work : new imperatives / Francis J. Turner.
    p. cm.
  Includes bibliographical references and index.
  ISBN 0-7890-0871-8 (alk. paper) — ISBN 0-7890-1596-X (alk. paper)
  1. Psychiatric social work. 2. Social service. 3. Social case work. I. Title.

HV689 .T87 2002
362.2'0425—dc21

2001039104

To those who have gone before
who still have much to teach us

# ABOUT THE AUTHOR

**Dr. Francis J. Turner, DSW,** was the first full-time faculty member hired for the inaugural year of the Graduate School of Social Work at Wilfrid Laurier University. He retired as Dean of the Faculty there. At various times he also taught at Case Western Reserve, Hunter College, and Oxford University and served in administrative posts. He earned his DSW degree from Columbia University.

Dr. Turner is editor in chief of the *International Social Work Journal* and has served on the editorial boards of a number of prominent journals. He has authored numerous books, journal articles, and professional presentations. Dr. Turner's work has been honored with many grants and awards.

# CONTENTS

# Chapter 1

# Introduction

The organizing thesis behind this work is that unless our profession turns once again to a broad acceptance of the concept and content of diagnosis as the heart of social work practice, we deprive our clients of a powerful helping resource and thus fail in our responsibility to them.

Although the project had been germinating in my mind for some ten years, it came to conceptual fruition one January morning in Cleveland during a snowstorm. I had just left Case Western Reserve University and was headed home to Kitchener, Ontario, about a seven-hour drive, when I discovered that the windshield wipers on my car would not work. I stopped at a nearby auto mechanic's shop seeking assistance. The mechanic on duty listened sympathetically and then informed me in all seriousness that he would not be able to tell me if he could help until he "carried out a diagnosis of the situation." His friendly professionalism conveyed an air of confidence. After about fifteen minutes, he reported to me both the good news and bad news, and what he would be able to do and with what level of assurance as to the prognosis for my next few hours of driving.

Here was an instance of the use of the term, concept, and application of diagnosis that was of considerable assistance to me as a driver. As I later thought about our conversation, it reinforced my long-held conviction that no one profession owns this term. It is a generic term that brings security to clients and practitioners in all professions.

Just two days after I had begun writing the first chapter of this book, the six o'clock news reported that during that afternoon a social worker in a distant city, in the course of making a home visit by herself to a single woman client, had been brutally murdered by this client. The client, according to the news broadcaster, was reported to have had a history of "mental upset."

Without knowing more about this tragic situation, I wondered whether this social worker had made a conscious judgment about her own safety in deciding to carry out this visit alone, or was she like so many social workers I meet who state they never make judgments or assign labels or diagnose?

Perhaps the question of her own safety, or lack thereof, had not entered her mind. Yet another possibility, one to which we must all pay heed, is that she indeed had carefully weighed all the available information and made the judgment that no risk was involved. It is important to know when a misdiagnosis has been made, for it then pushes us as a profession to ask if the deficit was in us or in a lack of available knowledge.

## Objectives

I have a threefold objective in writing this book. The first is to review the development of the concept of diagnosis in social work since it first formally became an essential part of the profession's lexicon. This occurred with the publication of Mary Richmond's book *Social Diagnosis* in 1917. The second objective is to put forward an argument that this concept's change in status over the decades from an object of pride to a pejorative word stems from a serious misunderstanding of the term *diagnosis*. This misunderstanding led to a sociopolitical conviction of the need for our profession to separate itself from terminology presumed to be the property of another profession. My third objective: I suggest that this reluctance to incorporate the term has had a negative impact on the profession and its commitment to accountability and, in so doing, has deprived clients of the quality level of service that we are capable of providing. If this point can be validated, then this discussion of terminology moves beyond the halls of academic debate into the realm of professional ethics.

The discussion focuses principally on those aspects of social work practice that emphasize direct work with clients—that is, that component of practice sometimes called casework, clinical work, micropractice, direct intervention, or therapy. This discussion does not presume a dichotomy in practice between large and small systems work. Rather, it assumes that social work practice, as it moves into its second century with the new millennium, represents a unified spectrum of theory, knowledge, and skills that cannot be divided. Certainly, the field of contemporary practice is so wide that individual social workers need to find their own specific component or components of the spectrum on which each will focus his or her attention, but this must never be to the conceptual exclusion of the total range of the profession's scope of practice. Thus, much of the discussion about diagnosis rightly focuses on one facet of the spectrum and is of less relevance to other components. Nevertheless, the conceptual basis of diagnosis—being understood as that process of a consciously formed series of judgments made during the life of a case, judgments upon which a practitioner bases his or her interventions, and for which each is prepared to take responsibility—does have application across all aspects of social work practice.

This matter of accountability is the most important objective of all. That is, it is interesting and important to understand how the term came to be a part of the profession and equally interesting and important to understand the history, politics, and sociology of the concept; the relationship of this change in terminology to practice is the heart of this project. Changes in a profession's terminology are bound to occur as we exist in a dynamic, change-seeking system. It is also expected that as a human service profession with a service element, unlike more abstract professions, our terminology will change frequently. However, as terminology does change, we have an ongoing responsibility to be vigilant as to the impact of professional lexicons on service.

I mention this need to be watchful as a form of self-confession. Although my early identification in the profession was with "the diagnostic school of practice," I moved to a wider focus on a broad-based interlocking theoretical approach to practice. In this growth process, I initially accepted the criticisms of others that the concept of diagnosis could be a limiting one for us and hence needed to be replaced by what was viewed as a less pathology, and more holistically based one. Therefore, although reluctantly, I did decide that the more politically correct term *assessment,* the one that came to replace *diagnosis* in much of North American social work practice, was acceptable. In so doing, both in my teaching and writing, I understood that this apparently greater comfort with the term *assessment* in the major practice textbooks was helpful, as long as it did not alter the practice concepts included in the term *diagnosis*—formal judgments leading to action.

However, in recent years, it has become increasingly evident to me that this shift in terminology was indeed more than word substitution. As I viewed practice, read case records in many settings, worked with clients, consulted with practitioners, and became involved in cases involving allegations of inappropriate social work service, I became more and more aware that as we moved to get rid of the term *diagnosis* we also seemed to be getting rid of the true meaning of diagnosis. I also became aware of the negative implications of this for practice.

As is discussed later, it appears that for a variety of very interesting sociological reasons, the term *diagnosis* was given a highly restricted meaning in the profession, one that emulated what were seen as the limitations of other professions. This misunderstanding and distortion permitted us to scapegoat the concept, legitimize our driving it out of the profession, and believe that by so doing we had "fixed" the deficits in our practice. We then saw ourselves as having achieved some type of maturational victory, which was presumed to ensure that clients were better served.

After long study, it is my conviction that the clients are not better served by the terminological change. Indeed, they suffer from it. Because of this, we need to readdress this discussion, and if my arguments appear to have validity we need to reinstate diagnosis to its rightful place of honor, the heart of social work practice.

I began this book, and the first draft of this chapter, out of a conviction that the term *diagnosis* had all but disappeared from the profession, apart from being alluded to as an interesting relic from our past. The basis for my argument was that it has clearly disappeared from the majority of social work textbooks. It has not only disappeared but clearly has explicitly been rejected by various authors. I will return to this in my later review of the literature.

However, as I talked about my interest in this problem to various groups as I traveled around, I found an interesting reality that contradicted what was being proffered in textbooks. What I found was that, indeed, many practitioners, for the most part senior practitioners, were very comfortable with the term and saw it as essential in their practice and discussions of practice. However, these colleagues were and are very aware that the apparent approved practice style was not to use the term. Its usage had been relegated to a form of underground vocabulary. Indeed, this reality that many in practice still viewed the term as important gave me further encouragement to address this matter in print. In the following chapters, I examine the place of diagnosis in social work and argue that it is important that we make it once again an essential part of our practice.

# Chapter 2

# The History of Diagnosis
# in Social Work

The history of diagnosis in social work is important, complex, and intriguing. It is important because its place in the profession's development is closely connected to our sociology and politics. It is complex because how it developed in social work has less to do with the concept of diagnosis than with other factors and struggles that made use of this concept to argue various positions about the nature and mandate of the profession. It is intriguing because it is a concept that has changed in a few decades from being the essential base of social work practice to being the object of scorn and rejection by many within the profession. As I examined the literature, I became aware that it is not possible to compact into a single chapter what is indeed an intriguing odyssey in our profession, one that deserves a full book in itself. What follows is a condensation of what in my opinion are the major components of this odyssey, with the understanding that my comments may not fully present the entire picture and certainly fail to mention some of the rich contributions of many colleagues over the years. What is evident is that a considerable body of literature exists that can serve as the basis for such an undertaking.

## *1920s*

Clearly, in attempting an overview of the development of the concept of diagnosis in social work, the starting point needs to be the publication of Mary Richmond's still famous, outdated, yet still relevant book *Social Diagnosis* in 1917. Here is not the place to analyze its place in social work history. This was done well by William Berleman on the occasion of its fiftieth anniversary in 1968 and undoubtedly will be done again on its centennial. For this purpose, I need only to identify that it is the work that in the sociology of the profession committed social work to a mission to base its activities with clients on a structured, testable, and accountable process.

For Richmond, diagnosis was the essential responsibility of a social worker. The process was viewed as highly structured, in which the social worker gathered large amounts of data about the client's personality, history, and social situation so as to come to a conclusion about the nature of the problem and the proposed structure of the interventive process. Diagnosis clearly was seen as a highly intellectual process and involved the assessment and categorization of each client. Richmond's (1917) formal definition of diagnosis was "the attempt to arrive at as exact a definition as possible of the situation and personality of a given client" (p. 51).

Diagnosis for Richmond was closely identified with casework and its tripartite conceptual base of history, diagnosis, and treatment. As a concept, it predated structured psychodynamic thinking and tended to be much more sociological than psychological in its presentation. However, it also had a strong research value orientation, a point that is often overlooked.

The much later view that diagnosis was more properly a medical term than a social work term had some of its origins in this early work. Much social work practice of the day dealt with public health issues and thus brought early social workers into closer contact with physicians and public health nurses than with other professions. Hence some, but certainly not all, of the early conceptual thinking was influenced by health concepts, including the understanding of the meaning of diagnosis. Richmond was adamant in insisting that her term *social diagnosis* was distinct from the term as used in other health disciplines and that other perceptions of the term *diagnosis* were not to be confused or interchanged. This idea was reinforced in her later book, *What Is Social Case Work?* (1922).

### 1930s

Literature about diagnosis seems to be almost nonexistent for the next ten or fifteen years after Richmond's writing. However, this may only show that I was not able to locate it. It appears that during these years the concept of diagnosis as a distinct and time-bound process that preceded treatment stood as the base for the teaching and practice of casework. Indeed, it was this close relationship to casework that in later years partially brought the concept into question.

In the literature of the 1930s that I was able to locate, there appear to be two themes, both of which are of current interest. The first is a criticism of a style of recording that seemed to be emerging in which emphasis was being put on verbatim accounts of what clients had said. This was being attributed to the impact of psychoanalytic thinking. The second theme is a resultant lack of adequate historical data from which a clear diagnosis could be made. Again, this demonstrates the idea that diagnosis was a fact and was time-fixed in the life of a case.

However, an interesting new concept is observable that began to address the process of diagnosis. That is, practitioners were becoming aware that as a relationship developed and as more material from the client's life was better understood, it was necessary to adjust, when appropriate, earlier diagnostic formulations (Finlayson, 1937). However, the theme from earlier days continued that the concept of diagnosis implied understanding the client's problems and their interactive dimensions. There was a strong problem orientation to the concept of diagnosis and treatment.

In looking at the proceedings of the early Charities Conferences of this period, it is interesting to observe that they were highly multidisciplinary, looking at issues, as mentioned earlier, of a public health nature such as nourishment, housing, safety, abuse, health, and poverty. Thus the papers presented came from a wide range of disciplines in which social workers played an important role. In this regard, there was much unchallenged cross-borrowing of concepts and terminology, including diagnosis.

Fern Lowry (1938) further developed the concept of diagnosis as a process and strongly criticized the trend to see history, diagnosis, and treatment as three time-sequential processes. "Instead of visualizing them as three portions of a straight line, we can visualize them as three strands of rope, interwoven from one end to the other, so that no matter at what point the rope is cut, we cut across all three" (p. 572). Diagnosis remained the essence of practice. Its definition remained the same: a thinking process aimed at deriving meaning. Lowry continued to see the term as generic to all professions and not the prerogative of any one. She used examples from engineering to support her views of its nature and definition.

A later article in 1939 by Taussig further criticized the idea of diagnosis as a one-time process and discussed how diagnosis can and should develop through the life of the treatment process and how all aspects of the process influence one another.

## 1940s

In the 1940s, I found a continuation of the development of the concept of diagnosis and an increasing understanding of its complexity and its interconnection with all casework processes. Authors were again underscoring the risks of separating processes. Charlotte Towle (1941) emphasized the interactive skill component of diagnosis and treatment:

> Diagnostic and treatment skills imply a capacity for precise analysis of a case situation into its parts, for comparative thinking of the parts in relation to the whole, and for synthesizing the parts into a comprehensive interpretive statement in which the essential elements of the case situation are still discernible and, therefore may serve as a treatment focus. (p. 458)

Later writings in the 1940s seem to move away from discussions of the nature and essence of diagnosis and toward the act of diagnosis, including the implications of the process for specific kinds of cases. The literature appears to take for granted the concept of both process and fact of diagnosis and emphasizes that as the treatment relationship develops, so too does the diagnosis change and develop (Simcox, 1947). In 1949, Hollis stressed the complexity of the diagnostic process and the need to take into account a wide purview of the client's life. There was no discussion of assigning labels (which emerged at a later date) but of attempting to understand the various dimensions of the personality and the situation of the client. It is clear in Hollis's writings that she was talking about a casework that is a form of therapy heavily influenced by psychodynamic theory. It appears that it was during the 1940s that the four concepts of casework, psychodynamic theory, psychotherapy, and diagnosis came to be seen as a unified concept. This perception later brought all four into question as various concepts were challenged from different perspectives.

These concepts were seen as a unified whole at the same time that much of casework practice was moving into family and mental health areas where many of the clients were highly motivated and where clients and workers perceived and expected treatment to be long term. This seems to be reflected in the literature on diagnosis, in which many examples were drawn from marriage adjustment problems. The stress here was still on diagnosis as a process of systematically understanding person and situation and on assessing potential for change (Sacks, 1949). In this literature concerning marital problems, a shift in the concept of diagnosis can be seen, from person and situation to person only. This is not a total shift; however, much of the discussion in the literature and many of the case examples focused much more on person, history, and inner dynamics than on systemic matters. Again, this reflects the strong influence of psychodynamic theory on the training of social workers of the day.

A related concern in the literature of the time was a growing criticism of the amount and style of recording and of the tremendous costs of the time it took to deal with it. Using voluminous recording as the basis of the formulation of a diagnosis rather than as a place to report it was criticized. This was connected to the style of supervision then extant, which had a component of using process recording as a basis for workers to understand their own dynamics in relation to a case. This, again, was a spin-off from the heavy influence of psychodynamic thinking.

### 1950s

In the decade of the 1950s, the themes already identified continued to predominate. In 1951, Hollis began to talk about psychosocial diagnosis rather than social diagnosis. In so doing, she began to identify that a part of the diagnostic process was to both "individualize and classify." The task of casework was to help persons learn to adjust more effectively to their social situations. There was very little focus on working to change situations. Diagnosis focused on trying to understand the sources of stress: Were they from within or without? But most of the focus was on trying to understand the total situation. Use of diagnostic syndromes, especially the understanding of the nature and function of neurosis, was often a part of diagnosis. Use of categories was appropriate, but practitioners were making a social work diagnosis that was in no way viewed as a medical diagnosis. Diagnosis and treatment were closely related and not fixed. Again, the idea of diagnosis as a process was stressed.

These ideas were also being challenged. Research showed that many clients only stayed a short time in treatment; thus diagnosis had to take place at intake. Short-term treatment was a valid concept and needed to be studied. An important theme that emerged is that in a diagnosis, practitioners needed to include more about the impact on persons of systemic issues such as poverty, neglect, and inadequate housing (Thomas, 1951). The term *diagnostic formulations* appeared to underscore the importance of seeing diagnosis as an ongoing process.

While the way to diagnose in particular types of cases was being discussed in the practice literature, the concept of diagnosis continued to be discussed in the theoretical writings of the profession. Gordon Hamilton's (1951) text, which was the basic teaching text in most schools of social work at the time, stated that diagnosis is "the thought process directed to the nature of the problem and its causes" (p. 24). Again, the focus was on the problem. She talked about diagnosis as a synthesis or interpretation of facts in order to give meaning. She emphasized that diagnosis was continuous, beginning with the very first impressions of the client.

In 1954, Lehrman continued the process of analyzing the concept of diagnosis, emphasizing that it was a "creative reasoning mode," and introduced the idea that diagnosis was similar to the process of hypothesis formulation and testing. He further emphasized that it was a highly complex process not to be considered lightly.

As the decade progressed, there was increasing use of the term *psychosocial diagnosis.* Also, the term *family casework* was discussed. This was not family treatment as it later emerged but a slight shift away from the idea that casework was one-on-one. Diagnosis was still highly identified with casework, however. Treatment was aimed at either maintaining adaptive patterns or modifying them, and diagnosis was related to one of these foci. There was still very little discussion of systemic changes.

During this period, the division between the diagnostic and functional schools was front and center. Aptekar (1955) said that both schools of thought diagnose, but the content is different. This identification of the later psychosocial theorists with the term *diagnosis* was the beginning of the minimization of the concept's significance in the literature and in teaching.

In 1957, Perlman addressed the concept of diagnosis and again underscored its importance. She indicated that the concept had begun to be challenged in the profession but stressed that, whether one is for it or against it, "every one of us is diagnosing as he relates to another person in a purposeful, problem-solving activity" (p. 165). She emphasized that diagnosis is the discipline that brings into conscious recognition a range of impressions and puts them together in a way that seems to make sense in view of our knowledge and theory. It is a process that is both intellectual and empathetic. She did not discount the complexity of the process but did reject the idea that a focus on diagnosis makes casework too intellectual, reminding us that it is a process in which we are involved in every human interaction.

Later in the decade as further theories such as systems, role, and problem solving were beginning to gain legitimacy in social work, there was less stress on the individual dynamics of clients of the earlier diagnostic school and more stress on a much broader view of clients in diagnoses. Special emphasis was put on family dynamics and family roles as an important area to include in diagnosis.

The complexity of the diagnostic process and the breadth of client and situation realities with which practitioners were involved engendered the possible need for social work typologies. This topic is still highly debated. Those against typologies argued that they led to stereotyping clients and a diminishing of spontaneity in practice. The other position was that such typologies would help give a more accurate focus to our practice and would ensure that appropriate systemic boundaries were maintained. Interestingly, some of the early attempts at developing typologies addressed the challenge from a problem-solving perspective. This concept that the essence of practice was problem-solving is perhaps the concept that has been most consistent throughout our history and has greatly affected the current view of diagnosis.

As the 1950s came to a close, we see an ongoing commitment to the necessity of diagnosis but a strong wish to greatly broaden its scope and its applicability to a broader range of practice situations. We see also the wish to incorporate the wave of new conceptual thinking that was emerging as the understanding and explanations of the psychosocial realties of clients expanded. In spite of this dramatic expansion, the vast majority of writings on diagnosis were still closely connected to the casework tradition.

In addition to discussions about the nature of the diagnostic process in the 1950s, there was a rapid expansion of literature dealing with social work treatment of various classifications of clients such as various physical conditions, psychiatric disorders, developmental stages, and ethnic, cultural, and class issues. Important as this was, there was also a concern in the profession that this type of literature fostered the idea that if practitioners could classify clients into one of these groups, they would know how to treat them. Out of this emerged the discussion of the use or harm of labels and typologies in social work, which sowed the seeds for the strong mistrust of the concept of diagnosis in the profession.

### 1960s

In the literature of the 1960s, it can be seen that the concept of diagnosis still retained an important position. Several of the themes from the 1950s were still prevalent. The first observation is that the concept of differential diagnosis held a prominent position (Turner, 1968). From this perspective, the literature is replete with articles addressing social work diagnosis and treatment of a wide range of different client types and problems including psychiatric categories, especially "character disorders," which were the special interest of social workers. Also, articles dealt with specific physical conditions and a growing interest in family issues. Of particular importance was the expansion of articles addressing sociocultural factors, a trend that had begun in the 1950s.

During this decade, group work was introduced in the clinical literature. Clearly, the concept of the multimodality practitioner was still only beginning. Articles discussed casework with groups and families, implying, but not saying, that these situations were different from the long tradition of group work and the rapidly developing family therapy movement. In this regard, the casework tradition seemed much more comfortable with the concept of family diagnosis and treatment and less so with the application of diagnostic thinking to groups.

A secondary theme, also a carryover from the 1950s, was the application of various theories to the conceptual base of diagnosis. Although rather short-lived as a theory that affected clinical practice, during the 1960s role theory had a high profile in schools of social work and in some of the writing about diagnosis. Two well-known colleagues wrote extensively in this area: Perlman (1968) and Strean (1967).

In an important two-part article, Perlman (1962) examined concepts of relevance to practice emerging from role theory and discussed their implications as a possible basis for a typology on which social workers could base a diagnostic classification scheme. Some of the discussions of role theory argued that it helped to put the "social" back into social work. This catchphrase emerged as segments of the profession were highly concerned that the development of clinical skills was focused on an aspect of the segments of society we were committed to serve that was too narrow and from a theoretical base that was too narrow as well. Looking to theories other than those with a psychodynamic base led to considerable reconceptualizing of the basic tenets of practice. Again, most of the discussion that addressed the issue of diagnosis was still taking place in the casework tradition.

As social workers struggled to broaden the focus of intervention, expand the use of differential methodologies, and incorporate the diversity of theories that were emerging as a part of a strong desire to be more autonomous, considerable interest developed in the concept of typologies of cases or problems that were proper to social work and that could serve as the basis for diagnosis (Turner, 1969; Finestone, 1960; Lehrman, 1960). As part of this search, attention was given to other categorical systems than the prevailing psychiatric ones, such as that published by the World Health. One of the concerns expressed by many was that as the knowledge base broadened, so too did the purview of factors needed to be included in a diagnosis. It was argued that if social workers could develop and utilize a classification system proper to social work, it would help them to communicate more effectively and thus contribute to the development of their knowledge base. One of the payoffs of a classification system that was envisaged would be an ability to record by code (Seaberg, 1965). This concern about recording was the ongoing reaction to the voluminous records prepared by social workers in the era of process recording.

Although there was considerable interest in the idea of social work typologies or diagnostic categories, there was more than mild concern that such categories would lead to an oversimplification of diagnosis and the possibility that diagnosis would be equated with the assigning of a category or a label to a client. Social workers had long been aware of the dangers of the misuse of labels, a concern that became more focused in later years. Although there was consensus that social workers did not aspire to assign a standard treatment to a given type of person, case, or situation, there was agreement that diagnosis was not an end in itself. Diagnosis was only of value if it helped clients achieve their goals.

Thus, in the 1960s, the growing interest in research was turned to the question of the relationship between diagnosis and treatment. Of great assistance was the work of Hollis, who had devised and tested a classification scheme that identified in a quantitative manner the various segments of an interview. This classification served as the basis for a large number of research projects and doctoral dissertations that examined various correlations between who the client was and what happened to him or her. Of particular interest was the question of clients' value sets and how they differentially influenced interview content (Hellenbrand, 1961; Mullen, 1969).

An ongoing theme throughout the 1960s was interest in and the need for increasing accuracy in diagnosis. There was considerable criticism of this lack of accuracy and the tendency to write imprecise diagnoses that said very little about the client and really could be said about almost everyone. Kadushin (1963a) wrote about this in a famous article, "Diagnosis and Evaluation for (Almost) All Occasions." Although it appeared to be a rejection of the concept of diagnosis, in fact it was an appeal to increased precision both in the formulation of diagnoses and the relationship of such formulations to treatment.

### 1970s

From the perspective of this discussion, the 1970s opened with an important article by Joel Fischer (1970) titled "Portents from the Past: What Ever Happened to Social Diagnosis?" He did a careful review of the history of casework in the profession and its move from a position of dominance in the field to one of lesser prestige. The discussion included the theme that while casework was seen as the preeminent method in social work, those who were designated as psychiatric social workers were seen as even more prestigious. Of course, this perspective included the identification with and stress on the importance of the concept of diagnosis. Since diagnosis was now seen as coterminus with a mental health orientation to practice, as the mental health orientation was challenged, so too was diagnosis.

Siporin (1970) argued that we need not discount the concepts of diagnosis and treatment but need to expand our purview of what these mean. He argued strongly for a return to and expansion of social work's concept of treatment to social treatment, which included the enrichment of systems theory and role theory. He argued that methods of practice cannot be divided. Social work needed to include individuals, families, groups, and communities in its view of practice. In this article, Siporin introduced the concept of assessment to describe a more holistic approach to diagnosis. Throughout, he took the responsibility to diagnose as given but saw it in a much broader perspective. Here the idea of diagnosis was separated from a single theory of practice and given a more generic perspective. Interestingly, in this discussion of social treatment the theme of problem solving remained dominant.

In the next year, Perlman (1970) continued the discussion of social treatment and social diagnosis. Diagnosis for her was no more or less than the basis of our design for action, that basis on which we *decide with the client* to move or not move in a particular direction. She too argued that diagnosis was not a term belonging to casework but to social work. Also, she argued that in diagnostic activities social workers need to pay much more attention to the clients, who they are, what they want, and what social work can offer to help meet their wants. She also reminded us that, as reflected in the research, much social work practice is short term but argued strongly that this in no way lessens the responsibility to diagnose. For her, the essence of diagnosis lay in questions of who a person is, what he or she wants, and what are the obstacles to achieving this want. Role theory and problem-solving theories were highly visible in this thinking, including the responsibility to judge whether problems come from within the clients or from their environment. Diagnosis is not simple in social work. There is a risk we can become so involved in the viewing that we forget the "doing." Diagnosis for Perlman was very much a process involving the client.

In 1972, Gelfand examined the extent to which the concept of social treatment had expanded into new fields, new theories, new areas, new uses of time, and new fields of practice. Although he did not talk of diagnosis as such, he did warn that social workers ought not abandon what they know in order to use their new understandings to build on the past. His underscored theme throughout was the rich expansion of ideas and knowledge taking place in the profession.

The theme of expansion rather than substitution of concepts continued. For example, Bloom (1973) urged social workers to return to more use of home visits to enrich their diagnoses. As yet there was no sense that social workers ought not diagnose but rather that they needed to enrich the basis of their diagnosis.

Scheunemann and French (1974) argued that diagnosis is the foundation of professional service but is not a one-time process. Rather, it must be ongoing and include the "assessment" of many aspects of clients' lives. Here we see the beginning of the use of the concept of assessment mentioned by Siporin, but so far it is clearly perceived as a process separate from diagnosis. Assessment is the process of deciding what areas of a client's life are significant in this situation and diagnosis the conclusions that permit us to start with a client, even though the diagnosis may change as the case develops and further assessments take place: "Diagnosis is always ongoing" (Scheunemann and French, p. 141).

Strean (1974) continued the understanding that both assessment and diagnosis are essential parts of the helping process. What is important in his writing is that he took for granted that social treatment includes individuals, groups, and families and that these modalities are called into play in relation to diagnosis, of which an important part is the client's wishes. He also emphasized the importance of a theoretical plurality as a new dimension to social treatment. In his view, this mind-set expanded the repertoire of resources available to the practitioner.

Throughout this decade, Hollis's writings continued to stress the importance of diagnosis. However, the focus of her writings remained casework, albeit a much broader perspective of casework than only one-to-one intervention.

A further interesting article on social diagnosis talked about diagnosis and the role that sociology can play in helping social workers to expand their purview in this area. The author (Chaiklin, 1974) argued that social work could be helped considerably in its complex activities, including diagnosis, by the development of more accurate typologies and stressed the advantage of interprofessional collaboration to help develop them. Social diagnosis was taken for granted; greater accuracy was emphasized.

In 1976, an article by Mackey appeared that stressed the importance of including the personality of the worker in the assessment and treatment process. What is important about this article is that it appears to be the first one that assumed that assessment is coterminous with diagnosis. In fact, the word *diagnosis* does not appear in the article. There is no challenging of diagnosis, just an assumption that the process of assessment is coterminous, as is evident in his description of assessment.

By 1976 the idea that diagnosis is principally related to mental health and mental illness had further concretized. An important article by Pruyser and Menninger (1976) discussed thoroughly the problems of terminology, nosology, and classification and the inherent risks of diagnosis for social workers. However, they concluded their article by insisting that diagnosis is the essence of psychiatric practice. Since during these years psychiatry was also struggling with the concept of diagnosis and its content, it appears that many social workers began to coidentify psychiatric diagnoses with social work's seventy years of tradition of social diagnosis. Since psychiatry was having the same problems with the content of psychiatric diagnoses as social workers were with social diagnosis, they must mean and be the same thing.

Scott Briar in 1976 analyzed in much the same way as Pruyser and Menninger on the allurements and traps of diagnosis. For him, social diagnosis is still essential to social work practice, not to get involved in the nosology disputes but to establish "a plan for action for and with the client." It is the basis on which we take responsible action. Diagnosis is risky but essential. In no way did he imply, nor did any of the other writers, that the term belonged only to other professions. Social diagnosis as an expanding concept belongs to social work and we must learn how to use it properly, avoid its risks, and enhance its accuracy with research.

The interest in typologies continued in the 1970s. Ogren et al. (1979) combined family diagnosis and crisis theories as a basis for a diagnostic system for social work. Like others, they built their work on the reality of the growing complexities in social diagnosis as theories and knowledge expanded. In developing typologies, they demonstrated how this process can avoid typing families and how it can maintain individuality.

Further work on the development of diagnostic models was taking place in England. Again we see further use of the word *assessment,* not as a movement away from diagnosis but as coterminous. The point was not argued in these writings; it seemed to be taken for granted (Hopkins, 1978). During this decade, Eric Sainsbury (1970) in England wrote an important book, *Social Diagnosis in Casework,* a volume that built on the assumption that diagnosis is a process essential to casework practice.

The coidentification of diagnosis with the so-called medical model and mental illness appears to have developed in the later 1970s as psychiatry was struggling with its own challenges in diagnosis. Social workers seemed to be writing less about diagnosis except in a critical way. Many social workers were identifying themselves with the anti-mental health-psychiatry movement, which of course strongly eschewed the idea of diagnosis, which was viewed as a commitment to labeling with all its supposed inherent evils. As social workers began to distance themselves from the so-called evils of mental health diagnosis, they also were being strongly influenced by learning and behavioral theory and its perception that diagnosis in a narrow sense is not needed (Wodarski and Bagarozzi). An interesting effort to develop a diagnostic typology for social work was made in a small volume written in Brazil for social workers in South America, titled *Services Social, Tipologia de Diagnostico* (Vaisbich, 1978).

However, the rejection of diagnosis as an essential part of treatment was not universal at the end of the 1970s. An effort to expand social workers' purview of its meaning continued, as mentioned earlier. As new theories began to impact on practice and practitioners, consideration was being given to how to translate new theoretical paradigms into diagnostic concepts of utility to practice. Keeney addressed this issue from what he called "ecosystemic epistemology," a theoretical approach beginning to strongly influence the profession, as it touched strongly on our long tradition of "person-in-situation." Inherent in this new approach was the strong idea that as theories develop, so too do diagnoses become enriched and practice enhanced.

## 1980s

In the 1980s, interest in diagnosis in the practice literature remained strong but not totally accepted. Those for whom diagnosis was an essential base of practice were placing more emphasis on the specifics of different aspects of the diagnostic process than on any discussion of diagnosis as an issue. In 1980, Carolyn Saari wrote about the importance of learning from linguistics to ensure more accurate diagnoses and how enhanced understanding of clients' usage can greatly assist in both diagnosis and treatment. In a similar vein, Harriette Johnson (1988) wrote about the need for accuracy in the diagnosis of borderline personality disorders. In this type of article, we begin to see very strong coidentification with the *Diagnostic and Statistical Manual of Mental Distorders* (DSM) (American Psychiatric Association, 1994) and the concept of diagnosis in social work.

The theme of this close relationship with the DSM continued through this decade. In 1981 Janet Williams urged social workers to become better acquainted with the DSM but pointed out that this is not the same as a social work diagnosis even though there may be common factors that demonstrate the importance of psychosocial factors in clients' lives. Later in the decade, Kutchins and Kirk (1987) warned social workers of the inherent risks of overdependence on the DSM. They addressed the question of the relationship between the use of the DSM and various forms of third-party payments that require a DSM categorization. Their overall conclusion was that the DSM is not good for social workers or clients, and they suggest we use our own discipline's body of knowledge as the basis of our diagnoses.

In an article the following year, these two authors reported on research into the use of the DSM by social workers and emphasized the need for social workers to be knowledgeable about it because of its very close connection to funding, but also again warned of an overdependence on it as the paradigm for diagnosis (Kutchins and Kirk, 1988). They took for granted that social workers need to diagnose but cautioned against a system that was principally devised for medical treatment. The next year, Elizabeth Anello (1989) responded to the two Kutchins and Kirk articles and defended the DSM as a useful adjunct to social work practice but only for certain parts of the profession.

In the 1980s, another interesting theme entered the discussion about diagnosis in which the possibility of social work diagnoses being made either by or with the assistance of computers was raised. It was argued that the process of social work diagnosis includes a series of decisions and thus should be able to be done by computers (Butterfield, 1986). A subsequent article by Nurius and Hudson

(1989) took this idea further and began to show some of the ways in which computers could assist in social diagnosis. As before, the responsibility to diagnose is taken for granted. It is the content, scope, breadth, and underlying theoretical orientations that have expanded to enrich the earlier idea of what is meant by social diagnosis, with the premise that the complexity of social work argues well for the utilization of computers. Examples of some emerging programs were given and social workers were urged to tap their potential for social work diagnostic needs and not to depend on other professions to do this for them.

As the decade closed, we see ongoing interesting discussions about the concept of social diagnosis and its place in the profession (Kirk et al., 1989). Here again the authors discussed the reluctance to use classification systems and hence social workers' ambivalence about the DSM. They reviewed again the history of the concept from Richmond's time to the present and stressed the contribution of the diagnostic model as developed by Hamilton and later Hollis. However, they urged social workers to develop their own systems of classifying clients and problems and mentioned the growing interest in the PIE (Person In Environment) system, which was then beginning to be discussed. At decade's end the commitment to diagnosis still remained important in the profession. The uncertainty that existed related to content and purview.

### 1990s

In this final decade of the history of diagnosis, we can see most clearly two opposing themes. The issue seems to divide principally along a textbook-versus-clinical literature parameter.

In examining the practice periodical literature of the profession, we see a continuation of the maturation of the concept of "social diagnosis" as the heart of clinical practice. The need to better incorporate multicultural issues in diagnosis was stressed by Solomon (1992). Interest in borderline clients as a common type of social work client continued in an article by Will Courtenay (1991) as well as the responsibility to make this component of the diagnosis accurately. In this article, although the term *diagnosis* predominated, the author seemed to correlate it with assessment. He thought that misconceptions and bias against diagnosis created the possibility that clients would be underserved. In 1992 Paula Caplan discussed gender biases in the way some DSM categorizations were made and the risks inherent in the misuse and biased use of some labels.

The difficulties and risks of coidentifying diagnosis in social work with the DSM continued to be a concern. Florence Kaslow (1993) introduced the idea of "relational diagnosis" as a way of expanding the base of diagnoses beyond the DSM. Social workers were urged to include more data about a person's history and pattern of relationships and to underscore that the nature of these diagnoses is biopsychosocial. In 1994, Turner argued that drifting toward the usage of assessment as coterminous with diagnosis is dangerous and results in a lack of precision and accuracy in diagnosing. In 1994, Carolyn Saari took a position that there is a clear distinction between the processes of assessment and diagnosis, seeing the former as a broad sweep of the client's reality and the latter as more specific, focusing on the immediate situation.

Ressler in 1994 introduced the concept of an ethical responsibility to accurately diagnose and based his arguments on the close relationship between diagnosis and treatment, pointing out the harm that can be done when the diagnosis is incorrect or incomplete.

Further discussion of the need to separate the concepts of assessment and diagnosis is found in a volume on dual diagnoses published by Drake and Mueser in 1996. The grand picture of assessment and the more targeted process of diagnosis are stressed in the various chapters of this collection. Diagnosis needs to be multifocused, and a consideration of the impact of various systems on a client's life is critical. The theme of the harm that can be done by inaccurate or imprecise diagnoses is repeated.

Other articles during the 1990s touched on the themes of accurate diagnoses built on the basis of assessment. These are two separate concepts that, although closely connected, need to be viewed as distinct. However, this emphasis on diagnosis changes quite dramatically in the methods texts commonly used in North American schools of social work in the 1990s. Overall, these texts include a strong antidiagnostic theme.

Zastrow (1999) stressed that the term *assessment* is preferred to *diagnosis,* implying they describe the same process:

> Assessment has sometimes been referred to as psychosocial diagnosis. But the term diagnosis focuses on what is wrong with the client, family, or group that is being diagnosed—such as

having a disease, dysfunction, or mental problem. Because diagnosis has a negative connotation many other social work educators, myself included, prefer the term assessment. (p. 59)

He later spends a lot of time on the nature of problems and identifying problems, failing to see that that is what he doesn't like about diagnosis.

Hepworth et al. (1997) wrote, "Historically, assessment was referred to as 'diagnosis' or 'psychosocial diagnosis' but we avoid the term diagnosis because of its association with symptoms, disease and deficits. . . . An assessment does include what is wrong, often including a clinical diagnosis" (p. 194). Again we see confusion about the term *psychosocial diagnosis,* meaning a DSM categorization.

Louise Johnson (1998), in talking about generalist practice, saw the two terms as the same: "The first step in the generalist social work process is assessment, historically referred to as diagnosis" (p. 265). However, she also said, "Diagnosis and treatment are terms that have strong connotations of medicine and illness" (p. 84).

Another well-known text by Kirst-Ashman and Hull (1993) took the same position: "Diagnosis focuses on pathology. What are the problems? What's wrong with the individual client? Assessment on the other hand targets not only the client's problems, but also the client's strengths" (p. 149). However, they do not appear to be consistent in that earlier in the volume they talked about diagnostic interviews as a separate type of interview.

Compton and Galaway (1989) also indicated their dislike for the term *diagnosis* because of their belief that it posits that "there is something wrong with the client" (pp. 474-475) and this is a decision made by the professional excluding the client.

The *Encyclopedia of Social Work* (1995) only refers to diagnosis in conjunction with the DSM and uses the term once in an article on managed care.

This interesting dichotomy between the practice literature and the textbook literature used in schools and faculties of social work appears to have created yet again a town-gown situation in the profession. As the generalist model of social work is seen as the prevailing practice model especially in bachelor of social work (BSW) programs, and with its strong view that assessment incorporates what has traditionally been divided into two separate processes, and with the accompanying perception that diagnosis is a negative term, it is understandable that the profession is less than clear about diagnosis.

In the 1990s, a further ideological movement influenced social work's purview on diagnosis. Postmodernism, the alleged new value base for social work, tells us that the concepts of diagnosis and treatment are carryovers from modernism, attachment to the scientific method and the medical model, and hence are to be avoided. To what extent this view will predominate in the profession is yet to be seen.

In summary, this review of the concept of diagnosis over the decades shows a much stronger continuity in its importance, nature, and content than I had expected in beginning this odyssey. In fact, it is still a critically important term for the profession. As with any concept, it has had to be examined, expanded, and modified as knowledge increased, theories multiplied, and methodologies expanded. At times, especially in the last two decades, it has strayed too closely to being coidentified with the DSM. It has also been identified with the needed search for social work categories of person, problem, and process. But throughout, the practice world has been strongly committed to the idea that responsible ethical practice depends on our understanding of who the client is, how worker and client relate, and how the worker can be helpful to him or her in an economical, safe, predictable way through processes for which the worker takes responsibility.

# Chapter 3

# What Led Us Astray?

Implied in the first chapter of this book is the thesis that we in social work have drifted to a position in which, for a large component of the profession, the long-standing tradition that held diagnosis to be the essence and core of responsible social work practice is no longer relevant. This project was begun with the perception that indeed the term was virtually moribund in current practice lexicon and of interest only for historical reasons. This conclusion was reinforced in an examination of the major methods textbooks used in North American schools and faculties of social work. As indicated in the previous chapter, apart from a few exceptions, not only are the majority of the currently used texts neutral about diagnosis give most the term a pejorative meaning and formally eschew it. This need to challenge the term intrigued me because, once I moved beyond the textbook component of our literature, I found that there was continued comfort with, and utilization of, diagnosis in the practice journals and articles.

I observed this same strong interest in the importance of diagnosis in talking to many practitioners and in consulting and lecturing to colleagues. What began to particularly interest me was the number of times colleagues and members of professional audiences took me aside after a lecture to "confess" that even though they knew it was out of fashion, they still considered diagnosis to be important in their practice and to thank me for restoring their faith. (I wondered at times whether in such situations I should assign them a small penance.)

In the original table of contents for this book, this chapter was titled "The History and Sociology of Diagnosis in Social Work." As I delved more into the literature and thought more about it, I concluded that such a title would be misleading, as I had not carried out a formal analysis of the available data in either a quantitative or qualitative manner. I suggest that it is a title and a topic that should be examined in more depth and comprehensiveness than can be given here. I leave it for other colleagues to address these two topics in a more scholarly and separate way. Nevertheless, I have long pondered the various factors that appeared to be operating in diagnosis's very vocal fall from "political correctness." In fact it was this curiosity that led to the decision to write this book.

Probably the two critical driving factors that led to the decision to address this question were as follows. First, I have always been and continue to be in awe at the skill of my frontline colleagues in their perceptions of their clients and the way that they engage in highly imaginative and effective interaction with them. That is, as a profession we are highly skilled diagnosticians. Over and over again as I hear colleagues talk of their clients, I am impressed with the thorough discernment they have of clients and of what is significant in the presenting situation for which clients have turned to a social worker. But of equal wonderment for me was that for the most part one learns of this diagnostic skill in talking to colleagues, certainly not in reading their records.

We are a highly oral profession. Over and over again I hear social workers present skilled, complex, and penetrating diagnoses of individuals, families, and groups that prove to be so accurate they appear to be a form of magic. Yet, in many of these same instances, a review of a case record would show little or nothing of this acuity. Since for the last twenty years in the teaching literature we have been insisting that social workers do not do social diagnoses, I began to wonder if this was an example of cause and effect. Assessments are plentiful, but frequently they seem to be brief (or indeed at times not so brief) social histories from which one has to guess at what was judged by the worker to be essential.

This reluctance to diagnose would not be of great concern if it had no other effects on practice. But in my view it does. One of the great challenges to our profession is to further develop our very rich body of knowledge. There is continuing and abundant evidence that we are highly effective with many of the clients we see. Our challenge now is to learn how to tap this store of effective practice to better understand who it is that we help and how we do it. That is, we need to find a better way of studying the correlation between diagnosis, treatment, and outcome in a manner that permits us to abstract data from thousands and thousands of cases rather than depending on the rich narratives of a few colleagues, important as these are. This gathering of knowledge is not intended to develop more books on theory. Rather, its goal is to find ways of helping more people, more quickly, and to pass this knowledge and skill on to those who follow us in the profession.

Thus, instead of this chapter attempting to parade itself as a comprehensive sociopolitical analysis of the place of a diagnostic tradition in the profession and how and why it has changed over the decades, I will only present my own observations with whatever distortions or omissions they may bring. Thus, in the following pages, I discuss the conclusions to which I have come as to why we have let diagnosis go astray. If there is validity to these comments, they may help us to once again restore diagnosis to a more visible and operational position in our practice.

I sensed the need for this chapter early in the process of planning this work, as I became aware of how strongly some persons in the profession objected to the term *diagnosis*. I had understood some of the concerns about it as we lived through a period of trying to make our practice more health and strength oriented and less pathology based, as diagnosis was purported to be. However, I soon began to sense that there appeared to be more to the issue than a preference for one term over the other, assessment over diagnosis. Rather, I began to understand that the term *diagnosis* has been made into a scapegoat by some within the profession. They could heap upon it, as in days of old, a number of concerns and then get rid of the concerns by driving it out of the profession like the goat going into the desert. That is, diagnosis had become loaded with attributed meanings and was used as club by some groups to assert a particular viewpoint.

As I will discuss in Chapter 5, diagnosis is a neutral term with very specific meanings applicable to the work of many professions. However, in the sociology of our profession, its neutrality seems to be long forgotten.

Several factors seem to be involved in its current place in the intrafamilial sociology and politics of the profession. As mentioned previously, its rejection by part of the profession seems to be partially related to a wish to change the profession, reducing an emphasis on what was wrong with a client in favor of a focus on strengths and potential. This argument was buttressed by a logic that said diagnosis is only a search for a problem or illness and thus needs to be eschewed.

This mind-set was, of course, also related to that period in social work development when we thought it important to shrug off any appearance of dependence on other professions, especially medicine. We wished to reduce what was seen as an overidentification with the field of medicine. Mary Richmond built her original purview of diagnosis on her close association with the health professions and we seemed to want to shake off this tradition. This was often expressed by calling upon yet another scapegoat, the presumed overreliance on the so-called medical model of practice in which a pathology perception of diagnosis was seen as an important component. Arguing, incorrectly, that this model (if it indeed ever existed as some presumed) was not interested in the strengths of people but only in problems, the model was thus to be rejected including one of its concepts, the responsibility to diagnose.

Thus the rejection of the term *diagnosis* was seen by some as a mark of our maturation. That is, if social work was to be an autonomous profession with its own body of knowledge and competencies, it must of course rid itself of any trappings of other professions. Although I can understand the wish in an earlier day for us to stand on our own, I have not fully understood why for many this term seemed to be most important to avoid.

This would be understandable if we did not use any language common to other professions and if we were consistent in this regard. However, social work, as one of the human service professions, of course has incorporated the whole lexicon of professional language into its day-to-day communications and writing including the word *profession* itself. Not only do we appropriately and comfortably make use of dozens of terms proper to any profession, we have indeed developed some of our own. These in turn have been adopted by other professions as part of the necessary and very helpful interprofessional cross-fertilization that takes place in multisystem structures. I think here of such terms as *casework, psychosocial, case management, biopsychosocial, counseling, task-centered therapy, problem-solving treatment, family therapy,* etc. These and many other social work terms are used comfortably by other professions with no sense of inappropriateness.

Another factor that seems to be part of this discomfort is more internal to our profession. I speak here of the ongoing concern in professional circles over the imbalance in what is called the micro-macro dichotomy. At different times during the past century, the profession was viewed by many as having turned away from sufficient interest in, commitment to, and attention to problem-producing systemic issues of devastating impact to our clients in favor of an alleged overstress on clients' inner psychodynamic structures. In these debates, terms such as *diagnosis* and *treatment* became symbols of this either-or perception of the profession and thus targets of criticism when this struggle was being waged in various professional arenas. Undoubtedly, the term *diagnosis* as it is commonly used in daily interaction in our society is probably more appropriate for smaller system work, even though it can be used very correctly in large systems of practice. However, as I discuss later, it is a concept with a much broader perspective than being a part of only the psychotherapeutic tradition of social work.

Another clear reason why in some circles diagnosis is unpopular relates to its close connection to particular theoretical orientations, in particular psychodynamically based theories. Since some, but certainly not all, of the important writing in this area did come from the psychiatric world, and since psychiatry was a part of medicine, this reinforced the idea that diagnosis was a medical term and thus not to be used by social workers. Also, since these theories did focus more on the inner person than the outer world, if this overstress of the dynamic was not understood they did shift attention away from the "person in situation."

As the profession began to struggle with the idea of a multitheory base, there have been many instances of intertheoretical holy wars. For a long time we practiced and taught from the conviction that one could practice only from a single theory. It followed that if one ascribed to one theory then it was important to show that other theories were wrong. Diagnosis was picked on as one of the psychodynamic terms to be rejected to bolster arguments for other theories. Fortunately we are in an exciting period when there is strong support for the concept of a multitheory base for practice, and there is much less emphasis on interturf theoretical struggles and more acceptance of the terminology of other thought systems.

A further component of the sociology of diagnosis appears to relate to the concept of power. Undoubtedly, diagnosis is a very powerful term, which can cause considerable harm to persons when it is misused, just as it can bring critically important, needed, and focused attention when accurately applied. Although in recent decades we have given considerable attention to the concept of empowering clients, there still appear to be segments of the profession in which there is much discomfort with our own use of inherently powerful ideas and strategies in order to empower. I have long found it of interest that, comfortable as we are with the need and advantage of empowering our clients, we seem at times very uncomfortable with the recognition and therapeutic use of our power to bring about the kinds of outcomes desired by the clients and ourselves.

Such terms as *treatment, diagnosis,* and *doctor* seem uncomfortable for many social workers. Let me comment on the title of doctor, again a title that in a very complex way has become identified in many areas of society with the profession of physician. We know it is a powerful title with many societal perquisites attached. One of the exciting developments in our profession has been the marked increase of interest in the social work doctorate and increase in the number of colleagues seeking this advanced degree. Many of our most gifted colleagues have shown themselves ready to spend the necessary four to five years of their lives in pursuit of this degree and the title it bears. What has been of considerable interest to me is the discomfort among many persons in our profession who have been designated as doctors by the same universities who grant the title *doctor* to psychologists, veterinarians, historians, philosophers, physicians, etc.

One can choose not to use this or any other title out of personal choices of self-effacement. However, in failing to use it in our practice, we deprive clients of the power that goes with the title, power that can influence access to resources as well as respect for, confidence, and willingness to invest in the services provided to them by us. Once again, we seem to incorrectly build into our perception and mores that this is a title reserved for only one profession. This reluctance to make use of potential sociological power and influence lessens our ability to influence the social systems we are committed to change in the search for social justice for all.

Clearly, this issue is tangential to my discussion of diagnosis. I mention it because I sense the same sort of internal dynamics may be operating that lead us to minimize our many strengths because of intraprofessional family disputes and debates. Similar comments can be made about our discomfort with the use of the words *treatment* and *therapy.* In these instances, we end up playing the same kind of word games, frequently substituting *counseling* for *therapy* as we do with assessment and diagnosis.

I believe a further aspect of this terminological issue is related to a misperception of the term *diagnosis* as having a unitary and fixed-in-time quality. Because of the broad spectrum of factors we need to take into account in seeking to understand clients in their biopsychosocial cultural realities, some believe that the term *diagnosis* is too restrictive to encompass such breadth and that the term *assessment* is more accommodating. As I discuss in the following chapter, diagnosis is not a unitary term in social work and does not consist of applying a restricted description of a client but can, does, and should have the breadth that is essential to our practice.

In beginning this work, I had somewhat presumptively thought that I would be the lone voice in the wilderness engaging in an almost quixotic mission. As the work has progressed, it has been of great interest to me to find that indeed the term *diagnosis* has not disappeared from our professional vocabulary. Rather, it seems that the difference in perception of this term and concept is more of a town-gown problem than a profession-wide problem. That is, if one examines the total spectrum of literature of our profession of the last few years, there can be found many references to and uses of diagnosis as a very matter-of-fact part of practice. The difference appears to lie between the textbooks of our profession and our periodical literature.

As mentioned, I began this volume after seeing time and time again in the important and frequently used textbooks for our methods courses in schools and faculties of social work a misdefinition of the concept of diagnosis used as a basis for rejecting it. With no proof given and in opposition to standard dictionary definitions, diagnosis is said to be a term proper only to medicine and to overstress problem and pathology rather than strengths. In a related vein, the term *diagnosis* scarcely appears in the most recent edition of the *Encyclopedia of Social Work.* Interestingly though, it is an item in the last edition of *The Social Work Dictionary,* where both the medical concept of diagnosis and the wider and more general connotation of the term are given.

One other area of note where diagnosis is considered essential to the profession is found in the legislation that governs social work in various jurisdictions. A review of this legislation in North America shows that in more than a few state and provincial laws related to social work, especially those that include a scope of practice definition, diagnosis is included in the legislated function of social work. Again, this seems to underscore what may be a factor of the sociology of town and gown.

As I continue to ponder this, the discussion that took place in social work of the different importance of qualitative and quantitative research comes to mind. This debate, for a short time, took on the trappings of yet another war of dichotomies in which one had to prefer one approach to research over another. Thankfully this has been resolved, and we are now beginning to see the advantages of each and the need to use both in our practice. In some way, the necessity for both assessments and diagnoses, and the distinction between the process and fact of diagnosis reflect the different aspects of qualitative and quantitative research.

One of the important developments in social work education was the very rapid movement from the MSW degree to undergraduate BSWs and community college teaching. With this very widespread development, of course textbooks were needed, and in the past twenty years a broad range of introductory methods texts have emerged. By definition, these texts are aimed at beginning students and practitioners and tend to seek a common core of beginning practice. In the same way, or indeed related to it, the wide spread of generalist thinking also focuses on core and beginning competencies, concepts, skills, and, interestingly, problem solving. I say interestingly because one of the major criticisms of diagnosis is that it is too problem focused. The concept of diagnosis carries with it a high level of responsibility and implied knowledge, which for many would not be appropriate at the undergraduate teaching levels. Since these texts take a strong position against the concept of social diagnosis, it is understandable that there is a basis for a negative position on this matter among many graduates.

In summary, without engaging in a thorough examination of the history and politics of the role of the term *diagnosis* in our profession, several themes internal to our profession appear to have impacted on the use and practice of both the term and the concept of diagnosis. These are more related to our internal development than to the essence of the concept. It is my position that this minimizing of the concept has also impacted on the precision of our practice, to the detriment of the clients we serve.

# Chapter 4

# Diagnosis: What It Is Not

My discussions of diagnosis thus far have reflected the firm position that over the decades this term has acquired a varied set of both narrow and incorrect perceptions in social work. This in turn has led to its being perceived in a negative way. Such misunderstandings still exist in many quarters and are handed on to generations of students, both in courses, as mentioned, and in many of the textbooks on which their professional formations are based. Also, these distortions of the term often serve as fodder for inter- and intraprofessional family feuds.

Semantic differences are of little import if they have no negative effect on the quality of services being provided to clients. However, it is my strong contention that this distortion of the word and concept of diagnosis does indeed limit the effectiveness of our practice by minimizing or discounting the richness, responsibility, and power of the term and the concept. Thus our clients are deprived of the benefits that a proper application of the concept carries in treatment.

I urge, therefore, a reevaluation of diagnosis in social work and a structured process of returning it to its proper position. As a first step, I suggest that we need to restore the term to our practice lexicon. To do this with conviction requires, of course, an understanding of what the term means. However, we must first understand what it does not mean.

## Diagnosis Is Not the Prerogative of Any One Profession

First, diagnosis is not the prerogative of any one profession. This is one of the most frequent mistakes made by our profession, and we seem to pride ourselves on our rejection of it. In its essence it describes the process of the series of judgments made by any professional that serve as the basis for taking or not taking a specific set of actions. Thus, in incorporating it into the lexicon of social work almost a century ago, we were acknowledging, indeed declaring, that as a profession we were prepared to take responsibility for our knowledge and for decisions and actions based on this knowledge. We understand well, of course, that as a human service profession social work shares much common terminology with other similar professions. Indeed, as a profession it should adopt the vocabulary that goes with professionalism, including such concepts as the word *profession* itself, as well as many others such as knowledge, research, skills, accountability, ethics, values, outcome relationship, intervention, treatment, skills, knowledge, practice theory, science, and on and on.

Of course, in incorporating terminology common to all professions, we must ensure that we take responsibility for such terms and give them our own meaning while staying within the generally accepted meaning of the term. That they will have common elements with the usages of other professions is to be expected and desired. In this way we can learn from one another and communicate with one another. But it is also understood that terms will have a uniqueness proper to our own profession. Both fortunately and unfortunately, Mary Richmond drew heavily on her understanding of diagnosis in medicine to formulate a concept of diagnosis for social work. She also, of course, drew concepts from law in her discussions of evidence and how to differentially understand it. However, this does not in any way lead to a conclusion that the assessment of information is only the prerogative of lawyers.

The important factor here is to distinguish the process of utilizing terminology, whatever its source, that is useful in enhancing effectiveness from the process of adopting it as a form of emulation or status-seeking. If we, or any group in society, decides that we must not use terminology that is common to other similar groups but must substitute our own, then of course we cease to hold a place among those groups designated as professions. This would create situations of potential confusion and discord, again to the detriment of our clients.

## Diagnosis in Social Work Is Not a Search for Pathology

Diagnosis does not describe a process in social work (nor indeed in any profession) that implies a search for pathology. Certainly the concept includes a responsibility to recognize problems and pathology when they exist. But equally important, the concept imposes an urgent responsibility to look for normalcy and strengths in presenting situations. This latter component of diagnosis is frequently over-looked by those wishing to discredit its utility. We greatly underserve our clients if we are interested only in identifying and responding to areas in their biopsychosocial situations that are abnormal or produce problems. As we are rapidly learning from a multicultural view of practice, if we seek only pathology it is highly probable that we will view many situations that are healthy and growth producing in a neg-ative way, especially if they happen to be different from our own unique personal value-focused view of the world. Hence the skilled diagnostician in social work (as in all professions) is constantly seek-ing to understand situations from a tripartite base, asking, what in this presenting situation is a strength in and for the client, what if anything is stress producing, and what about it do I not understand? Without a balanced perspective it is all too easy to overpathologize situations.

In a similar way, if we consider the word *pathology* or *problem* to be unacceptable, as they are for some of our colleagues, then we can miss critical areas in a client that are the sources of suffering and pain. We err grievously to view diagnosis as only a search for problems and further err when we believe and teach that this is what it means for other professions. Just this morning I had my annual (wife encour-aged) physical by my general practitioner, at the end of which he as-sured me that thankfully I was in good shape, apart from frowning at my caffeine intake. It is critical for this discussion to remember that the process that he went through to tell me this was just as much a di-agnosis emerging from a complex diagnostic process as it would have been if he had found something of concern.

### Diagnosis Is Not Solely a Search for Problem Areas in a Client's Life

In a similar way, diagnosis is not solely a search for significant problem areas in a client's life for which help is being sought. This is as important in contemporary practice when a "brief solution-focused" modality is in vogue as it was in an earlier day when "problem-solving theory" was the politically correct base of practice. Certainly many clients come to us who manifest a wide and complex variety of problems in their lives. In many instances, it is for these problems that help is being sought. As mentioned earlier, our skill as diagnosticians is to evaluate the strengths of clients and their ability to solve such problems, or to find solutions for them or help them find solutions in their own networks. But of critical importance as well is our responsibility to help judge with clients whether indeed they have a problem or not.

Frequently in practice, whether solution focused or not, our focus of intervention will be on helping persons recognize and make more effective use of their potentials, themselves, and their significant systems, with little or no emphasis on, or even knowledge of, problem areas. (Clearly we can get into semantic circles of little value here by saying that in such situations the problem was a client's inability or failure to recognize strengths.) Nevertheless, to view diagnosis solely as a process of problem clarification is a much too narrow view of this critical aspect of practice, one that fails to take into account our equally important responsibility to seek strengths and resources within the person's life that may offer opportunity for continued or enhanced biopsychosocial growth and functioning.

## Diagnosis Is Not a Process of Labeling or Categorizing

Related to the concepts of pathology and problem is the incorrect idea that diagnosis means assigning a label. Diagnosis, as viewed here and in most professions, is not a process of labeling or categorizing in a unitary sense. For many persons, it seems that diagnosis is viewed as the process of seeking to assign a label to a person, which in turn leads to either a particular form of intervention or a decision for nonaction; hence the term *diagnosis* is to be eschewed.

Most of us in social work have seen examples of this unifactor type of "diagnosis" made by our own colleagues as well as those in other professions and have rightly abhorred this practice. Indeed, one of the unfortunate spin-offs of this negative reaction to the use of a single label or category to describe a total person or situation has been the current faddish position that the use of any categories is unacceptable. I say unfortunate as it represents yet another example of the pendulum that has swung too far. Our position should be to resist the misuse of labels and rigid all-encompassing categories, not the categories in themselves. Categories and labels are useful, indeed essential, aids in communicating information, seeking precision, clarifying our thinking, avoiding mistakes in judgment, assuring appropriate interventions, calling into play specific resources, avoiding inappropriate interventions, and identifying areas of unclarity and uncertainty. It is impossible to communicate without the use of some kind of labels and categories. Thus, even to say, "I don't like social workers who label clients" involves the use of at least three labels.

What we want in the skilled diagnostician is the rich and skillful use of a broad range of categories and indeed labels covering many areas of a client's life. This helps us to bring precision to our perceptions of clients, to clarify where we are certain and where we are not, to identify areas of strength and limitations, and, of great importance, to specify areas where we require further information about the client, some aspect of his or her life, and existing resources or lack thereof. Of particular importance, we need to judge when we ourselves need help, either from one of our own colleagues or a colleague from another profession. Without a responsible and skilled use of labels and categories, diagnoses quickly become diffuse and imprecise and of little use to and for the client. What seems to be forgotten in the labeling dialogue is that when we try to get rid of one label, we have to find another one to substitute for it. Of course, there are times when labels should be changed, but the process is one of changing, not eliminating. However, when a term is changed the new term should not be a preexisting one that has a different meaning— for example, trying to substitute assessment for diagnosis.

There is a seductiveness to labels and their use. They can give us a false sense of precision and certainty, power and smugness. Thus in using labels and categories to describe clients and their life situations, we need to be aware of the degree of precision or lack thereof that is inherent in particular terminology. Also, we need to remind ourselves in social work that the purview of our clients and their network of significant environments is vast. This necessitates the usage of a broad range of categories, labels, and other descriptors as we seek to give ourselves, others, and clients a richer and hence more effective picture of how we view them as a basis for the actions we decide to take or not take with or on behalf of them.

In our appropriate and strongly justified concern about the misuse of labels, we need to keep in perspective that they are also powerful agents of help and reassurance. Recently I was told of a father, very concerned about his role with his young adolescent daughter, who sought out a social worker for help with his problem. What emerged from a single interview was a dramatic improvement in the relationship, which the father attributed to being told by the social worker that he did not have a problem; he had what the social worker labeled a very normal, healthy, typical fourteen-year-old.

## Diagnosis Is Not a One-Time-Only Act

Implied in the discussion of labeling is a concept related to time, best stated as follows: "Diagnosis is not a one-time-only act." One of the criticisms of diagnosis is that it is done once early in a case and stands as an unchanging basis on which all subsequent intervention is based. No profession views this concept in this way, and to do so is yet another example of a distortion of the process and the concept.

Throughout our history, social workers have maintained that this facet of social work practice, whatever it is called, is both a fact and a process that continues for the life of the case. It has always been understood that within the intricacies and power of the therapeutic relationship, both client and worker learn much about each other and mutually influence each other. From the social worker's perspective, this enhanced knowledge of self and other enriches the understanding of both strengths and limitations in the client and gives confidence in the manner in which the case is being handled. Or it may highlight uncertainties as to the direction in which the situation is moving. In most instances, as the diagnostic process continues, it leads to an enriching of understanding. However, it can also happen, and frequently does, that as we become more and more involved in a situation, we begin to understand that in fact we do not understand, and our diagnosis becomes less and less clear and certain. It is critical that we recognize such situations, for it is often then that we need outside assistance or additional resources that are beyond our scope. My own view is that one of the most critical diagnoses we make in practice is when we say, "I really don't know what this situation is all about and what I should do."

A review of our earlier history, when the process of social work intervention was conceptualized into the tripartite steps of study (or history), diagnosis, and treatment makes it evident that we then put undue emphasis on their separateness and perceived sequential characteristics. As a result, we gave insufficient attention to the more subtle and complex reality that these three abstractions describe processes occurring all the time in the life of a case. The very way that we greet a client in the waiting room, or wherever our first contact takes place, is a segment of our interaction, indeed of our treatment, and the client's response to us the beginning basis of our diagnosis. In a similar way the accumulating and formulation of our history, study, or information gathering, as this process has variously been called, often only begins after we have connected to the client in an enabling way, based on our initial diagnosis. I think we have frequently underestimated the high degree of therapeutic skill demonstrated by colleagues who are able to connect quickly with very complex and troubled persons in a manner that enables them to elicit the information needed to offer further help. Thus, in an interesting way, the actual time sequence of the therapeutic process, if indeed there is one, might well be understood as treatment, diagnosis, and then study.

It is important that we remind ourselves of the bureaucratic impact of much of the early mental health or medical social work practice that so influenced the conceptualizing of what was then called casework, which in turn became the basis of our first theoretical understanding of micro social work intervention. In a style of practice borrowed from the mental health field, practice from an administrative or bureaucratic perspective was built on the tripartite division of labor comprising first the taking of a history, second the formulation of the diagnosis, and third the planning and implementing of treatment. These facets of the helping process came to be seen as separate and distinct. Indeed, at times these activities were often carried out by separate persons. This perceived separation of activities then carried over into how social workers wrote about them and how we taught them to students.

Clearly it is easier to talk about and teach about such processes as separate entities than to address them in the much more diffuse manner of the interconnected, interacting, and interinfluencing reality in which they exist. Conceptually, it is appropriate and useful to address each phase of the complex process of professional interaction with clients just as we are doing in this volume from the perspective of diagnosis. However, the risk in doing so is overemphasizing differences and separateness and seeing them as time-fixed steps.

A further factor adding to this concept of a one-time-only action was the wish to simplify the emerging theoretical understanding of essential professional activities and to make them supposedly better understood by students and practitioners with little or no formal training in social work. In so doing, we greatly oversimplified concepts and gave them an inappropriate concreteness that failed to convey their complexity and interactivity.

Here I am emphasizing the concept of diagnosis as a process rather than an activity that occurs only once. Later I will also argue that diagnosis must also be a fact that is indeed visible and concrete. This is not a contradiction, for I will include in this argument that diagnosis is a concrete action that needs to occur several times through the life of a case rather than just at the beginning as in an earlier day. This to avoid the risk of an unchanging fixed concept of diagnosis or of over-emphasizing an ever-changing dynamic process. Exaggeration at both ends of this spectrum are dangerous. In summary, rather than seeing diagnosis as a unitary concept, it must be viewed as a duality comprising of both process and fact, where each component is of equal value.

### Diagnosis Is Not a Search for Status

A further criticism of the concept of diagnosis by those who choose to distort its meaning is that it is a search for status for the profession. It is not. Those who argue in this vein seem to think that social work has long aspired to receive as much recognition as of other professions, failing to realize that it already has long had such status. Indeed, rather than only being influenced by others, we have in fact influenced the practices and understandings of other professions. Since diagnosis is an important and respected concept to groups perceived as having this status, it will enhance our position to make diagnosis a part of our vocabulary.

No doubt in earlier decades, duplicating the qualities of other professions helped us in our growth and development. But there was just as much, if not more, commitment to do so from a wish to be accountable and effective as there was from a seeking of status by the insecure among us. Surely at this stage in our development, the motive of being fashionable ought not be an element in our selection of any terminology, be it useful or not. I argue that now that the period of needing to emulate the activities of other groups to enhance our own image is over, we should put away this habit of mimicry and utilize vocabulary that suits our own needs and those of the clients, whether it is also used by others or not.

When the idea and process of diagnosis are misunderstood, as many have and continue to do, it can rightly be viewed as a term that is not appropriate for what we do. Therefore, if it is a term that can harm our clients, then the argument correctly follows that we should get rid of it. But the need to overstress the challenges of diagnosis and its potential for harm appears to reflect that tendency of many in our profession to dichotomize concepts to emphasize their extremities. We clearly need to understand the risks inherent for clients in a misconstruing of the concept of diagnosis that supports a rejection of it. But just as important, we need to understand the risks involved in not stressing the correct meaning of diagnosis, risks that can have life and death implications for clients and others. We need to find a balanced position in this dialogue—*in media stat virtus,* as my undergraduate philosophy teacher used to say.

### Diagnosis Is Not Applying a Particular Theory

Although a diagnosis can and will be partially shaped by the theoretical basis of the person diagnosing, diagnosis is not in the seeking to apply a particular theory. Unfortunately, in the history of the profession the term *diagnosis* became attached to a particular purview of practice that was designated as "the diagnostic school." Hence, any use of the term is seen by some as a declaration of identification with this school of thought. This school, associated in its earlier days with such names as Hamilton and Hollis, was in turn viewed as being too dependent on psychodynamic and psychoanalytic theory. These theories and the practice models that emerged from them were once the heart of micro social work practice. However, as is the wont in our profession, this dominance was toppled and, as always, all went with it, including the term *diagnosis.*

For a variety of reasons, many of them valid, serious criticisms were raised within the profession of the tendency to view psychodynamic thinking as some type of absolute or to value it over other theories. Thus, as mentioned earlier, the reaction was in the form of the Hegelian antithesis paradigm, which is only now reaching its predicted form of synthesis. However, as we move toward synthesis, one which includes an acceptance that each theory has something to tell us and to offer clients, there is still a strong suspicion of concepts associated with this once powerful theory and practice model, and with it a suspicion of associated concepts such as diagnosis. Thus, in an effort to "cleanse" the profession's vocabulary, new words were sought, and not only new words but new understandings of the ideas that former words conveyed or presumed to convey.

Thankfully, social work has moved from a very naive theoretical base to a very broad one that has greatly expanded the repertoire of useful theoretical models available to us and hence to our clients. Many of these theories do include the concept of diagnosis. This is a tremendous leap of maturation. This comfort with diversity now includes a growing understanding of the powerful impact of psychodynamic theory as well as its continued usefulness, even though many are still suspicious of traditional things.

One aspect of this theoretical richness that is of import here is the question of diversity of terminology. In viewing different theories from the perspective of intertheoretical terminology, three things need to be kept in mind.

The first is that there are thought systems or theories that introduce new concepts and vocabulary into the profession's lexicon. For example, terms such as *equifinality* and *multifinality* from systems theory, are both new terms and new concepts.

Second, a new theoretical development introducing new concepts or interpretations of concepts may make use of terminology common to other systems. Thus, existentially oriented practitioners may emphasize the need for diagnosis but give it a much different meaning than do practitioners from other theoretical bases, e.g., ego psychology.

Third, new theories may use concepts from other theories without changing them. For example, crisis theory talks about such things as relationship, diagnosis, and treatment in a manner similar to ego psychology and psychosocial theories. Certainly these theories add new richness, insights, and dimensions to traditional concepts but within the framework of other theories.

In social work's tradition, diagnosis first was identified only with two or three approaches to practice. As new models of practice emerged, there was a strong tendency to alter vocabulary to argue for the import of some new ideas. Accompanying this was a tendency to criticize other existing theories rather than look for linkages between and among systems.

As I have examined carefully the similarities and differences across the at least thirty theories and models currently prominent in social work, I have not found any that lack commitment to a responsibility to attempt to understand the client in situation, out of which understanding the helping process emerges. Accompanying this is a commitment to taking responsibility for the process. This of course is my understanding of what has always been the meaning of diagnosis in social work.

It is hoped that in the next era of our development we will become more comfortable with diagnosis, so that our efforts can turn to understanding what each new theory brings to the enrichment of the diagnostic process rather than seeking new terminology to describe the process and having to sort out different meanings.

This discussion stems from a strong conviction that as we become more comfortable with the complexities of practice and our need to learn about and live with large areas of uncertainty, part of the diagnostic process will include two specific factors related to theory. The first is to begin to view theories as a treatment resources that give us different ways of understanding and intervening with clients. The second is the responsibility to include in our diagnostic process the question of what theoretical approach or approaches would be most helpful in particular presenting situations as well as which are counterindicated and could be harmful.

## Diagnosis Is Not Solely the Application of the DSM

As in the discussion of theory, diagnosis is not to be understood solely as the application of the DSM, in whichever of its many revisions it appears. This is not to be construed as a criticism of the DSM, a resource that has played a most important and positive role in helping to clarify terminology across professions, facilitate interprofessional expertise, and greatly enrich our understanding of the complexities and multifaceted aspects of various forms of human mental distress. This ongoing process of clarification, which is reflected in our comfort with change as knowledge expands, has resulted in clients receiving appropriate and timely help by means of more sensitive assessments and has limited the frequency of misassessment.

However, because of its popularity, its panprofessional usage and high status in recent years, it has come to be identified as the essential basis of diagnosis in the helping professions. This trend to make the DSM the heart and soul of diagnosis by equating diagnosis with a DSM description has been aided and abetted by many health insurance programs that provide coverage only for highly specified diagnostic classifications formulated in DSM terminology. This is particularly difficult for social workers, as we struggle with the complexity of our diagnoses, in which a DSM reference may or may not be useful.

Many of the situations with which we are confronted in practice do not and must not be looked at from the perspective of the DSM and its parameters, except of course in an exclusionary way when one makes the judgment that the clients do not fit into any of the many categories and subcategories described in the DSM. (It has already been suggested, of course, that if the DSM expands its categories any further, we will all fit into one of them, that is, of course, everyone but you, the reader, and myself.)

Just because many of the persons who turn to us for help are not DSM classifiable in no way relieves us of the responsibility to diagnose. We must remind ourselves that we need to make an essential judgment about the mental status of every client as we perceive it. This indeed is a diagnostic judgment! Thus, when we conclude that Mrs. Murphy is in good mental health and only needs help to manage her money more effectively, we have made just as important a diagnostic judgment as when we have judged her to be manifesting serious signs of depression requiring the assistance and diagnostic acumen of other professionals. To misdiagnose in either direction could have catastrophic consequences.

The DSM is a highly useful adjunct to our diagnostic responsibility. It has helped us to expand greatly our range of understanding of the manifest ways in which a person's mental functioning can get off track. But we err greatly as social workers if in any way we let it become anything more than a partial yet highly useful aid to our diagnostic endeavors.

### *Diagnosis Is Not a Clear Indicator of Treatment Strategy*

Inherent in the previous discussion of paradigms of problem functioning is an implied perception of a cause-and-effect relationship between diagnosis and treatment. That is, if I am clear about who the client is and my ability to help, there will be a prescribed way of working with him or her. That is, a clear and thorough diagnosis should lead to a clear, predefined, and thorough strategy of intervention or treatment. Probably this is one of the most critical ideas related to this discussion of what a diagnosis is not. It is my opinion that one of the most important maturational steps for the human service professions in general and social work in particular has been the growing understanding, appreciation, and indeed wonderment at the complexities of the interaction of persons and systems, which is the essence of our practice.

Two important concepts from systems theory are equifinality and multifinality. Equifinality is the understanding that similar inputs can have different outputs, and multifinality is the reverse, that different inputs can have similar outputs. These two concepts are highly relevant for us as they help us to avoid the perils of linear thinking. Such thinking leads us to believe that if one has a clear understanding of person and situation, one should also be clear as to the best way to achieve the desired outcomes. That is, similar precise diagnoses will lead me and my colleagues to similar patterns of intervention.

However, if diagnosis does not tell us what to do, then why should we diagnose? Isn't this very cynical thinking? Isn't our whole professional practice based on an assumption that to a considerable extent human behavior is predictable? We need not be overly concerned about this apparent lack of consensus that diagnosis A leads to treatment A in a lockstep fashion. Rather, this should humble us and reinforce our drive to look for patterns, to identify what helps when, and to gather data about effective and noneffective practice. Certainly there are emerging bodies of data that help us to understand what kinds of intervention help in what kinds of situations. We do recognize patterns of behavior and the types of reactions and patterns of behavior to expect in different situations. But this is far different from a diagnosis leading to a fixed prescription of intervention.

However, as we become more skilled and sensitive in our diagnostic endeavors, we should become much more sensitive and responsible to the clients, how they fit as interacting humans, and the range of resources and opportunities we can help them to draw upon or locate for them. That at some future date we may be clearer about identifying particular patterns of intervention that will respond to particular presenting situations is probable. At this point, we need to rejoice in our diversity and continue to seek ardently to be more effective in more situations, based on an increasingly accurate understanding of our clients and their situation.

## Diagnosis Is Not a Unidimensional Process

Neither is diagnosis a unidimensional process. This concept is alluded to in the discussion of labeling and categorization. However, because of the prevalence of an attitude that this is in fact what the term means, it is addressed here as a point in its own right. Many who oppose the terminology of diagnosis do so because they understand it as being very narrow in scope. That is, diagnosis is viewed as a process of identifying what is perceived as the major problem, disorder, or form of pathology which, once identified, becomes the target of intervention.

Of course this idea is attractive, as it gives a simplicity and neatness to the intervention process. Certainly there was a period in the profession's history that reflected this attitude. Earlier I spent some time on a search for diagnostic categories that would lead to patterns of intervention related to each category. This was thankfully short-lived as we became more understanding of the multiplicity of variables operating in clients' lives, more aware that our clients' lives were complex, and aware that the type of help needed was much more multidimensional than could be accounted for in simple diagnostic categories.

Unfortunately, this oversimplified search for specific treatment goals and patterned ways of achieving them was perceived as stemming from the terminology of diagnosis. Hence the term itself came into disrepute rather than seeing that it was being misunderstood and oversimplified.

Of course, one of the factors that assisted greatly in widening the purview of both diagnosis and treatment or intervention was the growing acceptance of the possibility, indeed the necessity, of viewing practice from an interlocking theoretical perspective, as mentioned earlier in this chapter. In a particular way, systems theory helped us to gain a basic and better understanding of how various components of a client's life interfaced and of how these interactions all needed to be taken into account in our diagnostic activities. It is understandable how attractive was the idea of a unidimensional diagnosis.

It is not certain that social work ever had a clear commitment to a unidimensional concept of diagnosis. The idea seems to be a form of overstatement in the often acrimonious disputes between various schools of thought. However, it is a position that some hold and thus must be listed as another of the things that diagnosis in social work is not.

## Diagnosis Is Not Done to or Imposed on the Client

Further diagnosis is not something that is done to the client or imposed on the client. Clearly, in an earlier day our perception of the diagnostic process did imply that the client had little say or input, especially in the era when diagnosis was seen as a separate process of decision making abstracted from the history or social study and upon which a treatment plan was formulated. Again, one of the dramatic payoffs of comfort with a multitheory approach to practice has been an increased and more sophisticated understanding of the complexity of the helping relationship and of our earlier naiveté about the implications of this complexity for treatment.

More and more we are coming to the understanding that the process of asking for help, sharing information, clarifying issues, formulating strategies, and evaluating our actions is a process in which the client plays an important and involved role. Increasingly, we are coming to understand that how we react to clients, how they perceive us, how they perceive the process, and their desired outcomes of the process are all parts of the diagnostic process, which, to be done accurately, must involve the clients. This broadened perception of the diagnostic process requires a change from the earlier idea that this was the responsibility of the clinician and indeed was something done to the client rather than with the client. Fortunately we are not the only profession that is facing this idea that the client and perhaps his or her family or significant others may be much more actively involved in the diagnostic process. Colleagues in allied professions are learning to do the same. Again, it is important that we understand that this is an enhancement of the concept of diagnosis, not a rejection of it.

In summary, it is my position that much, if not all, of the negative perceptions of diagnosis have resulted from a misunderstanding and misuse of the term rather than from any inherent defect in the concept. Diagnosis is a powerful term, replete with responsibility. It ought not be discarded because of its misuse, because in so doing we disempower our clients and ourselves. In particular, we ought not fear or avoid this concept because we perceive others to misuse it. Rather, we should insist on applying it to our own discipline in an enabling, powerful manner as an example to others.

# Chapter 5

# Diagnosis: What It Is

The previous chapter focused on a discussion of what diagnosis in social work does not mean. Although logically this present chapter should have been first, the negative material was presented from a conviction that the rejection of the concept stems from an overfocus on its misuses and abuses rather than on its essential and necessary meaning for practice. Such misunderstandings should not result in abandonment but rather in a commitment to reexamine it with a view to its reinstatement in a clearer, more accurate and precise way.

What then does the term mean for social work? Diagnosis in social work designates the process in which a professional opinion is formed stemming from the assessment of a situation as it emerges in our interaction with clients and their significant environments, an opinion on which we base our actions and for which we are prepared to be held professionally accountable. This professional opinion is based on a series of judgments that lead us to act or interact in particular ways with clients.

The essence of this definition is threefold:

1. Our diagnosis is based on the judgments we make.
2. Such judgments constitute the basis of our professional activities.
3. We are prepared to be held responsible for these judgments.

Because of our long history and a value position that we are "non-judgmental," many social workers are very uncomfortable with the word *judgment,* failing to distinguish the important difference between the two concepts. By judgment I mean the process of coming to a conclusion based on that critical mental faculty, discernment. It describes that constant cognitive and emotive process of evaluating situations in a manner that leads to action.

Being judgmental, of course, is much different. It refers to precon-ceived expectations or ideas, usually negative, about our interaction with others. It is a process in which we are constantly measuring peo-ple or their actions against some preexisting moral standard, values, or preferences.

Judgment is of course a powerful word; hence it is understandable that we may be uncomfortable with it. But we in social work must be-come comfortable with it if we dare to intervene in the lives of others. Whether we like it or not, or whether we seek to hide behind other softer words, in our practice we must and do continually make judg-ments that lead to action or nonaction.

Recently, after returning from the library where I had been work-ing on this material, I read two items in the national newspapers (August 9, 1998) in which social workers were being strongly criti-cized because they had made incorrect judgments in child welfare sit-uations. The criticisms were not that they had not made judgments, but that they had made incorrect judgments in areas where they were held by society to be competent. Such judgments led to incorrect ac-tions based on wrong diagnoses, actions from which grievous harm to children had occurred. That is, the diagnosis of each of these situa-tions was inaccurate. There was no criticism that judgment or diagno-ses had been made. It is important to remind ourselves that a decision to not act in a particular situation is, or should be, the result of a judg-ment. Indeed, it is also a diagnosis for which we are responsible.

One of the many factors that clearly distinguishes a professional re-lationship from a social one is the responsibility of the professional to seek continuously to be conscious of the judgments he or she is mak-ing throughout a presenting and ongoing situation. This need to dis-tinguish is essential because so many of the judgments required in a professional situation occur in the ordinary process of human interac-tion. We are so accustomed to this process that it becomes virtually a reflex, out of our conscious awareness. This is partially because it is very much a part of our day-to-day interaction with people. This bread-and-butter quality of human interactions thus easily gets carried over unrecognized into our professional interactions. The necessary skill of the social worker of making these interactions more con-scious is not easily acquired.

Throughout social work's history, we have expended considerable effort on the process of self-awareness. A great part of this process consists of helping practitioners become aware of their reactions to persons and situations of which they are frequently not conscious. What we have not emphasized sufficiently in this process is the need to help practitioners also become aware of judgments they make about people that are influenced less by their own inner dynamics or biases than by the human interaction skills acquired through their life experiences and sociocultural histories. Such judgments are of a different quality than the unconscious and preconscious material of our psychodynamic lives. But they, too, accurate as they are, lead to actions and responses to clients. These processes are the basis of our early and critical diagnosis of clients.

This concept of making critical judgments creates discomfort in many social workers, a discomfort that carries over to diagnosis. It appears to some that making judgments reflects a highly mechanistic flavor in our person-to-person interaction with clients or persons with whom we interact professionally, especially at a time when many new theories are urging a more humanistic and personal style of practice. The different interviewing and relating styles that have emerged from such theories are to be welcomed and endorsed, especially as they assist us in connecting to a much broader range of persons than do our more stereotypical psychotherapeutic modes. This conceptual position fits clearly with a commitment to seek to adapt our style or format of interacting with clients to a format that the client finds most comfortable. Our profession has long taught that our manner of relating to clients should suit the client, not ourselves.

However, even in the most informal or open style of interviewing, we are responsible for seeking to be aware of the conclusions or judgments we are making that lead us to respond in particular ways, seek particular information, move in particular directions, involve the clients in particular resources, connect with selected aspects of a client's life, or suggest particular methodologies. If we do not do this, we really are acting on impulse, routine, chance, or "gut reaction."

Of course, many times during the life of a case, particularly at the beginning, we do not know where we are with the client or where we are going in an interview. This is not so unusual. What is important is that we be aware of this uncertainty and consciously try to find a more understandable direction. I believe that one of the most important diagnoses that we make in social work is when we say to ourselves, "At this point I do not know what this is all about." Too often I fear that

our professional pride, often accompanied by bureaucratic exigen-
cies, pushes us to reach conclusions on which we take action inappropriately or without sufficient justification. Thus, as a part of our diagnosis, we always need to make a judgment as to our level of certainty
in regard to where we are going.

I remember clearly an event that helped me to understand this responsibility to be aware of our lack of clarity. I was practicing as a
young social worker in a psychiatric hospital. Several of us from the
unit were watching one of our patients, who had just been discharged
having greatly improved, walking confidently from the hospital with
her very pleased and welcoming family. She looked, and was, so
much better than when she first was admitted, and we were all feeling
quite pleased. The head of the unit, a psychiatrist who had taught me
a great deal, turned and said to me, "Well, Turner, have you or any of
us any idea how we helped that woman so much? I don't think we will
ever know!"

Of course one counterargument against consciously choosing our
style of interacting with a client relates to concepts of the use of
power. It is argued that I have no right to impose a style of interviewing on a client or to direct the content of the interview. Rather, my responsibility is to "start where the client is and let the client lead the
way as he or she wishes to."

While I am in total agreement with our commitment to work with
clients and to respond to them as far as possible where they are and
where they want to be, we also have a responsibility to help. This
often implies that we lead. It is naive in the extreme to think that the
client leads and we follow a form of dictum. We need to remind
ourselves that such things as the way we speak, the gestures we use,
our opening comments, what we look like, where we are, who we are,
and how we respond all influence "where the client is" and thus what
clients say and do. If we truly believe that an interview is a dynamic
process between two or more people, then to say that the client is the
one who directs the interview contradicts this.

As mentioned earlier, there was a time when diagnosis was seen as
a process that took place only after a prior process of history taking or
social study or investigation was complete. Also, it was something
that was done to clients rather than with them. Certainly one of the
exciting spin-offs of our expanded theoretical base is the idea of client involvement in the simultaneous processes of assessment, diag-

nosis, treatment, and evaluation. Many clients are their own best diagnosticians. For others, we can help in sorting out their situations, that is, in formulating their own diagnosis and when this is done they can, often much better than we, take over their lives with no further assistance. Frequently our function is to hear clients and validate their judgments about their own situations, that is, to empower them. At other times, it is our exchanges with clients that help them clarify where they are and what they should do. Remnants of this delayed and time-bound and "done to, not with" process still remain and serve to deter us from viewing diagnosis as both a process and a fact. In earlier days, diagnosis had a beginning and an end as a separate component of the interventive process.

Thus, as we come to better understand the intricacies and complexities of the professional relationship, we have learned with abundant clarity that diagnosis is a joint process. It starts at the very first contact with the client, indeed sometimes even before, and goes on through the life of the case and even after.

Although less formal than in our practice, in our daily lives we all make a broad spectrum of virtually instant judgments in any encounter with a fellow human. I address this spectrum of judgments in detail later. The point here is that not only do we make this spectrum of judgments, but we base our actions on them. As simple a thing as how physically close or distant we wish to be is the result of a series of judgments. What I want to emphasize here is that the diagnostic process begins much earlier than is often perceived.

Of course, I am not criticizing this very human process. Rather I am turning a perceptual searchlight on it. This ability is the essence of functioning in the myriad of human interactions that are part of our social lives. Our diagnostic skill in practice is based on our ability to make these judgments conscious so that we can test their accuracy, modify them in the light of subsequent insights, speculate on other alternatives, and assure ourselves that the resulting actions are appropriate. One very important facet of human interaction, such as that which takes place between a social worker and a client, is that it is *inter*action. Much as we seek to develop objectivity in our practice, each individual we meet impacts on us differently in a variety of ways, depending on who that person is, who we are, and who we are perceived to be. Thus, an important attribute of a sensitive practitioner in social work is awareness of our first and ongoing conceptual and emotional responses to a person. We can then ponder the accuracy of these responses and the need to modify them as the relationship develops.

I have given considerable thought to the best way to teach the matter of first contact with clients. The idea that we make a series of judgments about every human we encounter seems difficult for students. It seems to suggest overrationalization and distancing in a process they would rather view as more spontaneous and uncluttered. The language of judgments appears to carry only the image of a deliberative, rational, discursive process, which seems to detract from the exciting spontaneity of the human encounter. However, if we see this judgment process in a less cluttered manner, as somewhat similar to the hundreds, indeed thousands, of judgments we make about speed and direction, anticipated behaviors and actions when driving a car, flying a plane, or sailing a boat while at the same time listening to a ball game, talking to a friend, or preparing our next lecture, this concept is more understandable, humanly sensitive, and less daunting.

The range of judgments that need to be a part of any diagnostic process is discussed in a later chapter. One or two are mentioned here that are a part of our day-to-day interaction with our fellow humans to clarify the previous point. For example, although we are usually conscious of the process only in extreme situations, we all make a judgment about the potential risk to us when we meet someone. If we do not know the person, we also make a rapid assessment of his or her mental health, mental capacities, and score on our own internal desirability scales. I think as well that early in a first contact we make important judgments about a person's credibility and act thereupon.

Often our first impressions are very accurate and become more certain with time. But in our personal social lives we have all had experiences of being completely wrong, whether being too positive about a person or too negative. As mentioned earlier, for the most part, we are unaware of this complex judging process while it is happening. Only when something occurs to cause us to alter our first impression do we go back and ask ourselves, "How could I have been so wrong?" or "What was it about him that put me on my guard right away?"

Clearly, in our day-to-day lives we do not want to, nor should we, submit all of our interpersonal relationships to the type of analysis we need to do when wearing our social work hats. Probably all of us have heard someone say, often at a social event, "Now don't you start social working me." We must turn off our diagnostic and therapeutic miens, although sometimes we are not very successful. We have all had the experience of meeting someone who quickly involves us in an intense outpouring of some professionally laden material. At times it appears that we project an unseen aura that announces to others that we are social workers. However, we do need to become much more attentive to the process of judging in our professional interactions with clients and to seek to develop skills in making judgments conscious at an appropriate time as we continue the daunting and risky process of involving ourselves in the psychosocial realities of our clients.

It was mentioned earlier how quickly the process of driving a car can become virtually a reflex. However, as any of you who have taken defensive driving courses know, the major thrust of achieving higher levels of proficiency is to learn to focus on and make conscious your patterns of driving, the situations in which you find yourself, the abilities of the car, the condition of the road, the weather, and the anticipated actions of other drivers with whom you are interacting at say, sixty miles per hour. The purpose is to help us transform day-to-day driving skills, to which we give little attention, into consciously used skills to make us more safe, effective, and efficient drivers—to make us professional.

Diagnosis, then, is a highly rational process in which we seek to assemble our knowledge, impressions, data, information, and reactions to clients in a way that leads us to involve ourselves with the client in a particular direction, with a particular and identified set of techniques, strategies, and resources. This is done with the clear understanding that we and those we represent need to stand responsible and accountable for the appropriateness of these interventions.

It is implied that a social worker may decide to do nothing after a first phone call or interview. These types of short-term contact decisions are just as critical as the decision to move ahead in some form of extended intensive therapy. Their importance lies in their correctness, for a wrong diagnosis and a subsequent wrong series of actions can be disastrous, even life and death matters. I have often worried about settings where the first person to contact clients is a nonprofessional whose responsibility is to obtain an overview of the presenting situation and to decide when, where, and with whom a first interview is to be held. This seems to put an undue responsibility on our colleagues who are not professionally trained, for it asks them to make the initial critical diagnosis and to implement a brief treatment plan.

I am not suggesting that if we all agreed on the concept of diagnosis, our diagnoses would all be the same. This is not possible, nor indeed desirable, for several reasons. The first is the very important reality, which has been clearly understood and presented in existential thinking, that a part of the reality we need to consider in each case includes ourselves. That is, in our type of professional practice we are one of the significant others in a client's life, if even only briefly, and quickly take a place somewhere along the client's asset-deficit spectrum. We are a part of the amalgam, and thus an important part of our diagnosis needs to include a judgment about whether we are able to function positively in this situation, or an assessment of areas where our interaction with the client would be nonproductive. We need to be in practice only a short time to develop the powerful facility of being able to relate to the vast majority of situations that we meet. However, this does not mean that we can ever stop asking the question and making the judgment, "Is there anything about me or my actions that may be detrimental to my ability to help?" I suggest that as we become more experienced and supposedly more competent it becomes increasingly difficult to admit relationship problems in which we create the problem. I wonder how many case records have been closed with the comment that the client was not motivated for treatment when in fact it was something in the worker that was the problem. I think often of hospital social work situations in which we often found students in their first practicum being able to achieve great progress with patients and families whom we had despaired of ever being able to help.

Another reason why our diagnoses need not, and undoubtedly will not and should not, be the same stems from our growing multitheory base of practice. One of the distinct advantages of a multitheory base is that it gives us an opportunity to view cases from different conceptual perspectives. As yet we have not made full use of the opportunity for differential diagnoses that can result when we turn, as it were, different colored searchlights on a situation in a manner that might present us with new insights. These varying perspectives could well suggest more imaginative client-sensitive and effective intervention strategies. In fact a strategy which I suggest is greatly underused is to go through the process of diagnosis from two or three theoretical positions to see where we might find richer understandings of a case.

However, it would be wrong to overstress the idea that different theories will lead to highly different diagnoses. Certainly such diversity will result in different emphases on various parts of the client's reality, on the relative importance of particular personality factors, on the relevance of developmental issues, and on the differential weighting of external factors. On the other hand, all theories should lead to diagnoses that have much in common from the perspective of severity, risk, and potential. It has been demonstrated that each of the theories currently important to contemporary practice attempts to answer the same questions or to address similar aspects of a client's internal and external reality. They differ in the spectrum of responses to these items.

Probably the greatest differences between theories would be found in the identified treatment goals and strategies, their specificity, and the methods used to achieve them. However, whatever the theory, it is expected that such things as degree of seriousness, ability to function, capacity for growth, and potential risk to self and others would all be viewed at a similar level of intensity.

In summary, a social work diagnosis should mean, as it did for so many decades, the act of making judgments throughout the life of a case on those aspects of a client and the worker's ability to help them for which the worker is prepared to accept professional responsibility—and not some unitary search for pathology.

# Chapter 6

# Our Ethical Responsibility to Diagnose

It is implied in the discussion thus far that whatever our position on the vocabulary used to discuss the process, we all need to make judgments about clients and their situations. That is, responsible practice requires that we formulate a series of decisions based on our judgments of who the clients are, what is relevant in their lives in regard to their involvement with a social worker, and what of this will assist the worker to respond to them in a helpful way.

Often, when I talk with colleagues who deny that they diagnose, and even go further and state they do not make judgments, it is evident as they talk about their clients that they indeed have made a broad range of judgments about each client and situation based on an assessment of clients' personalities and their psychosocial realities. This statement stems from my observation of that interesting group of colleagues I have met who state they base their interventions on their visceral response to the client rather than on any cognitive process. Over and over again as I talk to such persons, I note how assuredly and indeed at times adamantly they will speak of clients and make summary statements about them in a manner that reflects a cognitive process. Thus, aware that many would deny this, I continue this chapter from the position that all who practice responsibly do indeed diagnose.

If we all engage in this process, why then *is* the question of ethics relevant? It is because of the earlier discussion of the distinction between diagnosis as a fact and diagnosis as a process.

As mentioned earlier, it is impossible to interact with another human being, whether in a social situation or a therapeutic one, without making a series of judgments and observations about them that shape our responses to them. Perhaps one could find exceptions to this in the most self-centered of persons who only view others as objects upon which they can vent and polish their egos, but such situations are the exception.

If indeed the process of assessment and subsequent judgment happens in all interpersonal interactions, then it becomes more essential in the interaction of client and social worker in a therapeutic alliance. But, as mentioned, in addition to this process of judgment formulation, there is the professional responsibility for the formulation of the "fact" of diagnosis. That is, not only do we make the judgments that drive our actions with clients, but our responsibility as professionals requires that we make these judgments known concretely to others.

I am not discussing the format in which the diagnosis appears. Since we live in a world of highly sophisticated and readily accessible technology, the diagnosis might be written, recorded, codified, computerized, etc. It is critical that there be an available external diagnostic statement or statements as a case develops about the bases for any action that is part of the social work process.

Why is this? Further, why is this an ethical matter? The general answer relates to our responsibility for accountability. That is, as professionals we accept the fact that our practice, confidential as it must be, is a process that can at times be scrutinized by others. Who are these others?

### The Client

As social workers we dare to intervene in the psychosocial reality of our clients. Such interventions can be highly critical, indeed at times of a life and death nature. Hence, our clients have a right to know how we have viewed them and how what we do with and for them is based on these perceptions. This of course is risky for us, as it may mean that our clients do not like what we are doing, are disappointed in us, or disagree with our diagnosis. But they have a right to know the judgments we have made about them, on which we have based our decisions to proceed or not proceed in a particular course of action.

### Our Colleagues

Our colleagues also have a right to know our judgments about a client and situation that have led us to proceed in a particular way. (I am talking of colleagues who have some direct connection to me and my work with clients and have some specific legitimization of access.) This is for a variety of reasons. First, from a collegial perspective, we should be able to assess the quality of work of those with whom we interact. This collegial responsibility is different from the administrative one, of which I will speak next. Rather it is our responsibility to one another of ensuring that those with whom we interact as colleagues practice in a manner that meets our reciprocal standards for one another.

We have a further reciprocal collegial ethical responsibility to diagnose related to questions of safety for clients, others, and ourselves. As mentioned earlier, many of the situations in which social workers are involved in contemporary practice deal with highly critical issues with inherent risks of violence and self-destruction. It is critical in the extreme that such situations are noted when they are judged to exist in the opinion of a social worker or a colleague. This is especially so if there is a possibility that a colleague may have to become involved in a case when the social worker is not available for consultation such as emergencies, illnesses, or absences from the clinical setting.

All too frequently in recent years, I have heard of situations in which violence occurred in cases where no fact of diagnosis was made out of a fear of incorrectly identifying someone as dangerous. These of course are the extremes, but the same responsibility exists in all cases to make our professional conclusions available to other colleagues who may have a legitimate right or duty to view them.

### Ourselves

For several reasons, we are ethically responsible to ourselves to record our diagnoses. Unless we are persons gifted with memories that can hold vast amounts of data easily and recall it accurately, there is no way that we can keep track of the essential aspects of our caseloads unless they consist of only one or two clients. Thus, to ensure that we can recall how we diagnosed a situation, it is essential that we record in some manner the basic components of the profile of judgments that we have made at whatever stage a case may be. We must ascertain what changes have taken place in how we view the situation as well as actual changes in the situation and respond appropriately. Also, we must continue the process of judging the level of certainty with which we proceed and when necessary continue a process of seeking greater certainty.

One area that must be watched of great importance is whether the client's goals and aspirations for the process have changed. Clients at times want to get out of a process to which they thought they were committed. Also, clients may want to go deeper and become involved in a much more intense process than when the case first began. Thus, a major component of the ongoing recorded diagnosis is to ascertain the degree of synchronization between the social worker's goals and the client's goals. This of course underscores the earlier point that the diagnosis cannot and must not be made only once. Rather, it is a process of regular reconsideration of all aspects of a case to ensure that we perceive and understand changes that may or may not be taking place and to respond accordingly.

## Our Setting

Similar to our responsibility to our colleagues, we also have a responsibility to our setting to record a diagnosis. A component of this responsibility is similar to what we owe our colleagues to ensure that clients receive optimum care and attention and that colleagues are alerted to the gravity of situations when we are not available.

However, there is a further level of responsibility for the agency, to assure from an administrative perspective that clients are receiving quality intervention in relation to available resources and that such intervention is based on clear diagnoses by the therapist. In a practice setting it is important to know the kinds and distribution of the clients who are served, who is helped, who is not, what resources are needed, and what patterns of service exist in relation to the mission statement of the setting.

Important as this information is for the internal life of the agency, often there are also external bodies such as funders, accreditors, and government departments to whom the setting may be accountable. In such situations, administrators must know who is being served, how, with what outcomes, and with what certainty.

## The Profession

Responsibility to the profession is perhaps more abstract than the previous ones but nevertheless is real. The development of knowledge in our profession is based on an ongoing assessment of what it is that we do with and for which people and with what outcome. Certainly, some such knowledge is gained through research, which is separate from the analysis of direct practice of which I speak here. However, the largest source of new knowledge must be the study of what we do, why we do it, when we do it, to whom, and with whom or for whom we do it and what happens when we do it.

That we are highly effective with many of our clients has been sufficiently demonstrated over the last two decades that we can be comfortable about our overall effectiveness. What we lack now is a clear and precise understanding of whom we help and whom we do not help. We need to find ways of increasing our effectiveness in measurable terms with various kinds of clients, problems, and situations. We need to be able to better assess the different impacts of various strategies and techniques. We need to understand better the differing utility of our application of helping theories. But to progress along this long and tedious road of knowledge building we need to have available to us a much richer coterie of factual diagnoses so that we can better understand the bases on which social workers act and with what outcomes and thus compare different uses of knowledge and technique.

Over and over again, I view agency records in which it is evident that the social worker involved was of tremendous help to the client, but in reading the record I have no way of knowing on what basis this help was given. If one talks to practitioners, they can almost always give a rich diagnostic profile of the client and the situation. That is, the process of diagnosis exists, but the record is lacking.

### The Public

We also diagnose for the public. As with our responsibility to the profession, there is a related responsibility to record our diagnoses for the public. *Public* here refers to those other components of society who at various times and in various situations have a legitimate need to scrutinize our practice, including such groups as accrediting bodies, certain public bodies, the court and legal system, disciplinary bodies of our profession, researchers, and students. I recognize, of course, that this right is highly restricted and should only be granted with the greatest of care and concern.

Nevertheless, we have learned in recent years that even though we may wish to keep all our records confidential and only between us and the clients, this is not always possible. Courts and our colleagues rightly need to know in various circumstances the judgments we have made. To not record these decisions is viewed rightly by society as a serious omission or fault, as when we unfortunately have made wrong decisions.

However, it would be unfortunate if we viewed our records only in a negative sense. Frequently, we can be of tremendous assistance to our clients when we present clear, precise, authoritative reports and descriptions about them that include our diagnostic decisions in regard to our actions or recommendations about some aspect of their lives or the lives of significant others. This is especially important when we are seeking a particular type of service for them.

In summary, we are increasingly coming to realize as a profession that ethical social work practice includes a commitment to both the process and the recording of diagnosis. We are not yet at a point in our knowledge and practice where we have consensus on the format of the records.

Until we have the opportunity of examining many hundreds of diagnoses, we need to be comfortable with such diversity. The ethical issue at stake is that there should always be available to those who have a right to it a statement as to the judgments about a client that served as the basis for the decisions made and the actions taken during the various stages of the intervention. I raise the matter because of the very high prevalence of case records that show no evidence of a diagnosis, or even if the term *assessment* is preferred, such assessments lack data on the critical professional judgments made at various relevant points in the case.

# Chapter 7

# Our Ethical Responsibility to Label

It is impossible to talk about the art of diagnosing without quickly getting into a discussion of the use of labels. I begin this chapter on the assumption that we have moved far beyond the social work parlor game, so popular a few years ago, that attempted to divide the profession into two groups, the pro- and antilabelers. What I used to find so interesting in this dialogue was that those purporting to see labeling as evil could bolster their arguments only by the application of labels. The statement "Surely you are not one of those social workers who labels clients" includes at least three labels: client, social worker, and label.

I believe that most of this debate took place in the hallowed halls of academe. The presumed politically correct position of several years of students was to be against labels. However, most practitioners understand that it is impossible to talk about a client without the use of labels, recognizing, again, that the word *client* is a label.

Nevertheless the debate was worthwhile, for it helped us to focus on and clarify several areas of practice. The first was the terrible harm that could be done to a client by performing a diagnosis by assigning a single label describing some aspect of the person in situation from some glossary or other; for example, "Charlie is a schizophrenic"— end of diagnosis!

The second thing that we learned was the harm that a label could cause when inappropriately applied. That is, as we came to appreciate the power for good or evil of particular diagnostic labels, we were reminded of the terrible responsibility to use them carefully and to check their accuracy frequently.

We also learned the risk of having a concept of diagnosis as a fixed process that once formulated is to stand for ever. Most of us know of young children to whom labels were assigned as part of their diagnoses, and who retained these labels for years as if the labels described fixed and unchanging aspects of their situations even though they matured.

We also came to understand better that many labels, although originally viewed as benevolent and useful in intent, take on a popular, imprecise, and frequently pejorative meaning and thus need to be changed. The word *retardation* is a good example of this. The term emerged to replace the word *idiot,* which originally also had benevolent conotations. In its original intent, retardation meant someone who was delayed in development. This earlier term might actually still be more precise than *developmentally handicapped,* which replaced it and which already has been replaced by the shorthand DH. There are many more! Hence a part of the watchdog and gatekeeper function (two labels in themselves) of any profession, especially social work, is to be alert to the popularizing of terms in a distorted fashion and to work on a process of reclassification when this happens.

Thus the debate about whether to label or not to label was useful but oversimplistic. Most important, it helped us to understand that it was not labels we were against but rather

1. the misuse of labels, and further the misuse of certain labels;
2. the translation of the label to the whole person;
3. the inappropriate stigmatization carried by some labels; and
4. the need to seek new labels when one has become distorted.

But I suggest we learned an even more powerful lesson. That is, it was just as dangerous to attempt to practice social work without a labeling process as it could be to overuse labels with all their perils:

- To deal with a client who is clearly suffering from some form of schizophrenia from a position that one should never attach that label to a person may result in that client not receiving a rich repertoire of resources that would be of considerable help to him or her.
- To fail to understand that omitting from my diagnosis a judgment that a client is seriously paranoid out of a dislike for the term may result in me or a colleague being killed.
- To not accept that the label of autism can open the door to a rich range of resources for a family is unethical in the extreme.

- To not include a label of political refugee in my purview of a client may completely miss the essence of a person's current crisis or difficulties in adjusting.

It is unacceptable to play games when we know, for example, that a person is seriously mentally ill, suicidal, or violent and we attempt to avoid stating this by substituting other, less precise words or euphemisms. This is an avoidance of responsibility of the worst kind. However, in using labels we always need to keep in mind that frequently such labels are very imprecise in themselves. As we know, a term such as *schizophrenia* is a good example. However, even though much is still not known about this condition or conditions, the term does convey sufficient clarity to give us some understanding of behavior and some indications of strategies of intervention and helpful resources.

Obviously, in assigning categorical terms we may be wrong and at times will be. But this is how we learn, and in such cases we need to ask why we were wrong. To not make the judgment out of a misguided commitment to neutrality of language is equally worrying. It can cost you, the client, or others their lives at one extreme and lack of access to helpful resources of person, technique, and material at the least.

A critical component of the use of labels is the grave responsibility to make two further judgments about any label we use in regard to a client. The first is to attempt to quantify an observation, if it relates to a quality or characteristic that lends itself to quantification. Thus, it is not sufficient to state in a diagnosis that Mrs. Murphy appears to be depressed without stating as well how depressed we judge her to be. There are depressed states that would lead us to take a client immediately to a hospital emergency room and other levels of depression that are real yet so mild that clients can continue to function quite well on their own. Over and over again I see the phrase, "The client appears depressed," without any indication of the severity or lack thereof. The same holds true for another expression frequently seen in records: "This client is anxious." Again, this is a state that probably applies to most of us some of the time, but it also can be so severe that it is totally immobilizing.

A helpful strategy in the process of quantification is to think of the characteristic under scrutiny on a scale of one to ten and decide how to rank the client. We need descriptive vocabulary to reflect this quantification such as mild, moderate, severe, critical, etc.

Another aspect of the use of labels is that we should include in the process and the record some indication of the level of certainty with which we are making a judgment. This again is highly important, for it leads us to move with caution or comfort or somewhere in between. This aspect of judgment also leads us to seek further data, or when necessary to seek another opinion in critical situations. When we are uncertain or when uncertainty is high, we move with much less assuredness than when we are clear and certain. This lack of certainty argues again for the idea that a diagnosis must not be fixed. However, the need to record a diagnosis periodically pushes us to test in a concrete way our certainty and clarity in each situation.

It is much easier to talk about our responsibility to label than it is to be clear about the vocabulary and terminology that best suits social work. Inevitably this discussion raises the complex question of areas of responsibility of different professions and what kinds of terminology are acceptable between professions. There is a technical issue here, for in different jurisdictions some groups are excluded from making what are viewed as medical diagnoses and thus the sole prerogative of the medical profession. However, this is different from a social worker presenting a professional opinion: I suggest that it is appropriate for a social worker to state in a diagnosis, "In my judgment, Mrs. Murphy is exhibiting mild schizophrenic tendencies." This is very different from stating, "Mrs. Murphy is mildly schizophrenic." This matter of what we can say or not say in a formal diagnosis is a long way from being clear and will vary from jurisdiction to jurisdiction. But this does not excuse us from our responsibility to state clearly our view of who the client is, to quantify such judgments, and to state our degree of certainty about them.

It is implied in the discussion of quantification that the variables in which we are interested are always negative and of a symptomatic nature. Not so! As is discussed in Chapter 7, the areas of a client's life about which we need to make judgments are broad. This breadth makes our diagnoses much different from those in other disciplines. Thus, we are interested in such things as the richness of a client's social network, the strength of significant relationships, systemic influences, the integrity and richness of personality characteristics, the availability of material resources, the level of satisfaction in a diverse role set, and on and on through the gamut of judgments that need to be a part of our diagnoses. Many, perhaps most, of our diagnoses will use none of the hundreds of labels available in current mental health lexicons, and from the perspective of a client's mental functioning will say nothing more than "in apparently good mental health." The critical thing is to make a conscious judgment about this area, initially and through the life of the case, including a decision regarding our level of certainty.

I think it useful to remind ourselves that the decision regarding labeling was settled for us many eons ago. I believe it was in the book of Genesis where Eve and Adam were given the task of assigning a name, "a label," to all the birds and beasts. I think a process that started so long ago is not going to be undone by some scholarly debates to the contrary.

One of my very real concerns about colleagues who say they do not use labels is that they then do not include some critical judgments in their assessments. I think this can happen very easily in settings where most of the clients are in good health both physically and mentally, so that whether judgments of these aspects of the clients' reality are made or not is of little consequence, because for the most part these are not important factors. However, it is because most often health is not an issue that practitioners need to make such decisions in each case, for it is the ability to pick up on those very few instances where mental health is an issue that separates the responsible worker from the mundane colleague. Society and the profession expect us to be alert to and aware of the extraordinary aspects of a case. If we only dealt with the ordinary, there would be little need of our training and body of professional knowledge and skills.

In summary, it is the thesis of this chapter that not only must we engage in the ongoing process of diagnosing, but we must ensure that in recording of this process we strive to put clear labels on the aspects of the presenting situation we have judged to be the basis on which we proceed in a particular direction with the client. Indeed, in my view it is impossible to write a responsible diagnosis without the careful and judicious use of labels.

# Chapter 8

# A Spectrum of Critical Judgments

Previous pages referred frequently to the judgment component of diagnosis and the need to make judgments as specifically and consciously as possible in each situation. To achieve a high level of objectivity and consistency, it is important that we base our practice on some type of template or paradigm of factors. In the last decade, I have sought to develop such a paradigm by identifying those judgments that need to be made in each social work case situation and arranging them in a format for use by practitioners.

Although I have not as yet tested this template through formal quantitative research, I have continuously attempted to refine it through qualitative processes, an ongoing study of social work theories, and the reading of many cases. I have now reached a point where I have not made many changes in it in the last few years, and I am comfortable in putting it forward both as an aid to practitioners and as a basis for comment and critique by my colleagues.

The template has been developed as a form of aide-mémoire for practitioners. It could also be used as a paradigm for diagnostic activity, and I hope that this will be done in the near future to further test it. The following pages address the major components of this outline and reasons for the inclusion of some of the items. The most current draft of the template is included at the end of this chapter.

The first section addresses those judgments that we need to make, however tentatively and however potentially imprecise, to justify continuing or not continuing with a case beyond the first contact, whatever our theoretical base of practice and whatever the setting. As mentioned earlier, many of these judgments, especially those related to our immediate interaction with a client, are made in the very first few minutes. They are gradually refined, corrected, modified, or expanded as the relationship develops and some form of helping process is instituted.

The first group of items (1 through 7 on the diagnostic checklist, page 82) are judgments that I suggest we make about every new person with whom we come in contact. Because these decisions are so critical and so much a part of our daily lives, they become virtual reflexes in our interpersonal functioning. For the most part we are not aware we have made such judgments, unless we consciously focus on them, except in extreme situations when they become very evident to us.

Since these judgments are so often unconscious, we seem to forget that they are critically important judgments that we also make about our clients, and they affect the way we interact with clients, from the first contact. Thus our diagnostic responsibility is to learn to consciously address these items in each case, our degree of certainly about them, and of course their implications for a continued relationship with the client.

I suggest that one of the very first judgments we make in an interaction with a new client is related to personal safety. The accuracy of this judgment can have life and death implications. However, we are aware of this judgment only in extreme situations when safety seems genuinely threatened. Our tasks as practitioners are to learn to first make these judgments more conscious, and to make them sooner and more accurately than would the general public.

I well remember one day walking down the hallway in the school of social work past a partially open door of a colleague. On seeing me, she called out and asked me to join her in an interview with a very well-dressed, controlled, well-spoken young male student who had dropped into her office for information ostensibly about our social work program. (We later decided that it was a well-disguised cry for help.) My perception in a very few seconds was that I was in the presence of a very hostile, highly disturbed, and highly dangerous person. My colleague had judged him in the same way; hence her decision to quickly involve someone else, who happened to be me. Further discussion with the young man confirmed our diagnosis, and together we were able to get him in contact with available mental health services. Our original judgment of the emergency nature of the situation was confirmed, and very effective help was provided.

As practitioners, a further judgment we need to make early in a contact with any client is whether clients are a risk to themselves. As we know, suicidal thoughts are sufficiently prevalent among our clients and when overlooked can lead to tragedy. Of course, most of the clients we see are not suicidal or even close to it, but because some are we must consciously judge. What I find most distressing is that in many cases workers have not even considered suicide as a possibility and miss those rare situations of very desperate but highly veiled cries for help.

In a similar way, we need to judge the risks to someone else. I am not suggesting that there are large numbers of clients who are going to harm others. I am saying that it is a real possibility for some of our clients and it is our task to consciously consider this possibility rather than take our chances on levels of probability. What saves us from serious situations is that, apart from highly specific types of settings, the vast majority of our clients are not going to be a threat to others in their lives. But we need to remember that society does not pay us for ordinary day-to-day reality but for our ability to respond appropriately and quickly to highly idiosyncratic situations.

In our interpersonal interactions, we also make immediate judgments about the level of a person's intelligence. This is manifested in such things as the way we alter our vocabularies, the content of our speech, the speed at which we speak, etc. These shifts in relating and communications are so automatic that, apart from the extremes, we are usually totally unaware that we have made them. Making ourselves aware of these judgments pushes us to ask the further diagnostic question, "Why did I make this judgment, and were my data accurate in so making it?" I have often noticed that we can make serious mistakes in our first assessments of a client's intelligence based on accent or dress or particularly visible physical limitations, such as a speech difficulty. When we make such judgments incorrectly, the whole interpersonal process of further contact with the client can be seriously skewed.

Without getting into the debate as to whether social work diagnosis implies a DSM classification, a part of the first cluster of judgments about a person includes an assessment of his or her mental status. Even if we cannot spell psychiatry or have never heard of the DSM, we all make a judgment of a person's mental functioning and act or react accordingly. Sometimes in our nonprofessional interaction, we move as quickly as we can out of the person's presence; at other times we quickly judge that here is a well-integrated soul mate with whom we can interact in a pleasant, comfortable manner. The point here is to remind ourselves that:

1. We do make such mental status judgments.
2. We need to be aware that we make them.

3. We need to assess our degree of certitude about them.
4. We need to assess how our judgment is affecting the present situation.
5. We need to determine whether this effect has relevance for our diagnosis of the situation.

In a similar way, we make very quick and (as we mature) accurate judgments about a person's communication skills, basic personality characteristics, basic value set, and level of credibility.

In summary, I contend that a conscious review of our judgments of others is essential to all social work diagnoses. Because they are so automatic, we frequently fail to incorporate these judgments into our diagnosis of a client. These judgments affect our style of interaction with people, the content of our discourse, our levels of comfort, the nature of the role we enact with them, and our general disposition toward them and thus are critical to the diagnostic process.

Our challenge as social workers is to understand that we have made the concept of diagnosis much too narrow, failing to perceive that our decisions in these identified areas are the driving points of the subsequent style and modality of our professional interaction. This is difficult because the first-level profile of judgment discussed here probably are made within two or three minutes of an interpersonal interaction, or even less. As we get comfortable with this idea, we find that our ability to get along with people is highly related to our skill and speed in making this profile of judgments. As social workers, we become highly skilled at this, to the point where we frequently are not aware that we have engaged in this process. But this fact does not obviate our responsibility to review of this process objectively to test the accuracy of our judgments, to identify when and where we have been wrong, and to ensure that we work at enhancing our accuracy. Again, as mentioned earlier, our professional responsibility is to take this very human process and skill and hone it to a level beyond the norm.

I have put particular stress on this initial component of diagnosis because of my experience of reading many social work records over the last three decades, which has shown that the worker has made a series of important judgments about a client but with no indication of whether the worker is aware of the judgments he or she has made.

In addition to this cluster of human interaction judgments, in any social work practice situation there are other clusters of more professionally oriented judgments we need to make about clients that affect our ongoing work with them. None of these will be a surprise to the reader. It is just that so often case records contain only descriptions and assessments of various aspects of a client's life but no indication of what conclusions or judgments the worker has made as to their relevance to the case.

One area that we seem to frequently overlook is the client's overall physical condition. Of course we are not attempting to function as physicians. However, we know from our own lives, from our professional experiences, and from various theoretical bases that a person's overall health affects many areas of his or her psychosocial functioning, either temporarily, for example, a person with the flu, or on a long-term basis in someone who is in chronic pain or discomfort. Our responsibility is to be aware of such possibilities and to take them into account in our overall judgments.

Of particular importance in this area, and in our North American society, is our responsibility to know something about the client's use of medications. As we know, a large percentage of our population makes use of various forms and combinations of medication. We also know that many of these medications affect a person's overall functioning in many ways, either temporarily or on an ongoing basis. Again, our task is not to attempt to function as pharmacists or physicians but to be aware of the possibility that medication is part of a person's life and to ensure that we obtain the necessary knowledge about its possible effects when it may be a factor in the person's functioning and presenting situation.

Most of the other items on the checklist are diagnostic areas that social workers commonly address in their work with clients and need only some general commentary. My position is that we need to separate the process of assessment and diagnosis in each of these areas. In so doing, we need to focus on three questions: (1) Do I know anything about this area of the client's life? (2) Do I need to know anything about this area? (3) If so, what is its significance in the presenting situation? In many instances, we know very little about many areas in a client's life; indeed, we may not even know a client's name. My position is that we should constantly keep before us that profile of information that may be relevant and be aware of areas in a client's life and aspects of a client about which we have sufficient information to make judgments and those that we have consciously judged not to be relevant.

One of the risks of suggesting a paradigm such as this one is that it will push us back into a practice of gathering large amounts of information about each client before we make any decisions and take any actions—the old days of the long and involved social history. This is not what is being suggested. I propose that it is our responsibility to be aware of the many aspects of a client's psychosocial reality that we may need to look at and make judgments about in order to function responsibly. But also, be aware that in few, if any, situations will we ever have a complete assessment of all aspects of a client's life. Our skill as practitioners, especially in this era of short-term interventions, is to learn how we can act responsibly and effectively with a minimum of data.

Clearly, we want to be driven by the law of parsimony, that is, to learn to function with a minimum of intrusion into a client's life. But we must never forget to be aware that we will meet highly complex and high-risk situations where we can indeed be lifesavers based on our ability to assess accurately the interfacing of many areas of a client's reality and to respond to these complexities in a growth-enhancing, empowering, enabling way.

A couple of areas on the checklist ought to be underlined specifically, ones that in my reading of records most frequently seem to be overlooked. One of my concerns over the last few years, as many of the practice texts and much of the short-term literature have focused on problem solving of various types, is that we tend to overlook the concept of strength. Over and over again in records and forms used by agencies, stress is put on the identified problem or problems. Clearly if a client has a problem, and I stress *if,* we need to understand it from the client's as well as our own perspective. But we need to formulate a diagnosis from the perspective of strengths both in the client and the client's significant environments of people, systems, and resources. Many case records give the reader no indication of the strengths in the situation but only focus on the problem.

For example, a preliminary diagnosis might read as follows:

> The presenting situation involves a single father expressing concerns about his relationship with a teenage daughter. In my opinion, he is a well-integrated, highly intelligent, well-motivated single father with a large network of helpful family and

who needed only professional assurance that he was doing well and need not be seen again.

Another situation might be considerably different:

> The presenting problem is a single father expressing concerns about his relationship with a teenage daughter. In my opinion he appears to be highly anxious, with little understanding of his role and few family resources, but a strong wish to be an enabling father. I believe he will need an initial short-term but intense relationship to help him become more self-assured, followed by a group experience where he can learn about the role of single fatherhood.

That is, in each situation we need to identify the conclusions or judgments we make about what is going for us in this situation and about which and what concerns us. In addition to helping us properly judge a situation, an inventory of role, personal, material, systemic, and interpersonal resources can be therapeutically enabling and empowering to clients.

Related to the question of strengths is a possibility that I think we often overlook, which is to ensure that we judge whether indeed a client has a problem or not. I realize that the very fact that a person comes to a social worker could be interpreted as meaning that he or she has a problem. I am more and more convinced that we are seeing more than a few people in our society who only want the opportunity to look at some aspect of their lives or to talk about some existential component of their reality with an understanding professional. To say that such people have a problem is, I believe, a misuse of the idea of problem. In fact, seeking us out ought rather to be viewed as a strength in that they find they can best review their lives in interaction with a professional. I suggest it is totally wrong to have to classify such persons according to some problem list in order to serve them, as we do in some administrative structures that are built on the basis that our work is essentially problem solving.

Another important facet of our diagnoses, which I think we need to address more frequently, is to ensure we understand and then compare what the client is expecting and wishing to get from the relationship and what we perceive is needed. Frequently these two perceptions will be congruent but at times could be very disparate. For example, in my view, we may be convinced someone should get out of a particular relationship, when what he or she wants is to find a way of living more safely in it. It is critical, and I suggest, often missed that without clarity of these two therapeutic goals, our work with clients may be of little help to them. This awareness of a difference between what the client wants and what we think would be helpful is not a new theme in social work. It is raised here in relationship to diagnosis to ensure that we ask the question through the life of a case and build it into our judgments about the process as it develops. Of course we need to be aware that objectives change in both client and practitioner, and such changes need to be noted in the process and record of diagnosis.

A further judgment we often forget to include in our diagnosis is our perception of the client's motivation. Just because clients have come to us does not mean that they indeed want to achieve their stated goals. Levels of motivation change throughout a client's life. Indeed, one of our important therapeutic roles is to enhance, support, foster, and at times help create motivation. I suggest that an important component of our ongoing diagnostic process is to make regular judgments about level of motivation.

In addition to level of motivation, we need to ask ourselves what judgments we have made as to our overall level of certainty of our diagnosis. Of course, the sociology of professions pushes us to argue in support of our diagnoses. However, I suggest it is most helpful to the client and to us to periodically ask ourselves about our level of certainty in general and in particular components of a case. This certainty often fluctuates through the life of a case, and thus it helps us to consciously consider it to focus on both why we are less certain at some point in a case and to work to clarify such uncertainty either through our own efforts, in conjunction with the client, or in consultation with someone else.

Related to our level of certainty is the discipline of attempting to prognosticate about where a case is going. Again, this is a topic not frequently addressed in the practice literature. However, it is a component of diagnosis that aids our conceptual understanding of particular case situations and our knowledge in general as well. I think we gain the most knowledge in situations where we have been wrong in our prognosis. That is, we anticipated a particular outcome for a case, which turned out to be incorrect. Frequently this is not a negative. Cases often move much more quickly than we thought they would or a client's life changes much more dramatically than we would have ever expected.

Of course, the reverse is true in that some cases turn out in disappointing ways. In all cases of unanticipated outcomes, an important part of our diagnostic responsibility is to ask, What did I miss here? What strengths were present that I failed to properly take into account? Or, conversely, What weaknesses did I miss or what resources of knowledge, technique, or service did I misuse or underuse? Humbling as this is for us, it is also an important way to learn.

I think as a profession we would gain much by developing some type of tradition similar to the medical postmortem. In such a process, either as individual practitioners or as colleagues, we would periodically examine a case following its termination and seek to identify in a learning but not critical way what we did correctly in relation to our diagnosis and what could and should have been done differently.

In summary, the theme of this chapter is that we fashion and hone our diagnostic skills by developing a continuous process of examining and making explicit the ongoing process of judgments that are a part of any human interaction in a general way but are much more targeted in our profession.

I am uncomfortably aware that the process I am suggesting here can be viewed as detracting from the spontaneity of any human relationship and converting it into a highly cognitive, cerebral one. We are only in our profession a short time before we begin to appreciate our skill and the satisfactions we gain in being able to relate quickly, empathetically, and helpfully to the broad range of the human family with which we interact, regardless of our practice setting. We know that in the intensity of a close relationship with a client, which may involve the most critical life situations, little of our conscious attention is given to the judging process. My thesis is that our skill and responsibility in practice is to bring to consciousness the judging process that is going on all the time.

Spontaneity and the cognitive process of making accurate judgments are not mutually exclusive. Indeed, they are mutually enhancing. The spontaneity becomes more accurate and sensitive as the judging process becomes more concrete. This ability to combine these two skills occurs in many professions. Earlier I mentioned how drivers become highly skilled through their ability to understand the thousands of judgments made in a few minutes of driving on a busy highway. Ordinary drivers make the same decisions and judgments almost without awareness. What makes the trained driver more skilled is his or her ability to understand what and why such judgments were made. As social workers, our task is to work assiduously at building our interventions on a rich range of judgments, understanding that the more skilled we become at this, the richer will be our interventions in the lives of our clients.

## A Diagnostic Checklist

Following are the areas to be considered in making the series of judgments required in formulating an ongoing assessment and diagnosis. The format presumes a single client and thus needs to be adjusted when the client is a dyad, family, or group. In assessment, we seek to understand these areas in a client's life; in diagnosis we formulate a judgment as to what, if any, significance they hold in this presenting situation.

A.

    1. Overall mental status
    2. Intelligence
    3. Safety
       a. In relation to therapist
       b. In relation to others
       c. In relation to self
    4. Basic value set
    5. Basic personality characteristics
    6. Communication skills
    7. Credibility

B.

    8. Overall physical condition and status
    9. Medication
   10. Significant role set
       a. Roles
       b. Adequacy of role performance
       c. Comfort in role set

11. Cultural, gender, racial, ethnic, and religious factors
    a. Identity
    b. Significance
12. Significant others
    a. Strength
    b. Quality
    c. Availability
13. Significant social systems
14. Significant impinging history
15. Substance use or abuse
16. Interpersonal network
    a. Strength
    b. Quality
    c. Availability
17. Major strengths in
    a. Persons
    b. Significant environments
    c. Resources
18. Major problem areas, if any, in
    a. Persons
    b. Significant environments
    c. Resources

C.

19. Perceived needs
20. Client's wishes and expectations
21. Perceived nature of service to be offered
22. Required availability of help
23. Present level of motivation
24. Prognosis
25. Overall level of certainty

# Chapter 9

# Diagnosis As a Process and a Record

Throughout these pages I have warned against falling into a semantic trap in which we view diagnosis in a unitary, concrete, fixed fashion. Unfortunately, as discussed earlier, for many, both the professional and popular usage of the term reinforce this idea of singularity. However, as we begin to clarify its place in contemporary social work practice, its dual nature of both process and record quickly emerges, and this duality needs to be held constantly in view to properly understand its implications for practice.

## *The Process*

By process is meant the professional responsibility of gathering, analyzing, classifying, weighing, pondering, ordering, questioning, and judging that begins when we first take responsibility for a case, be it an individual, couple, group, family, or community, and is ongoing through the life of the case. Although over the decades we have used terms such as *history* or *social study* (but no longer *investigation* as in Mary Richmond's time) as if they were discrete entities, we know that such a perception only poorly reflects the process that occurs when a human being interacts with a professional in a therapeutic way. As mentioned earlier, the very manner by which we greet clients may be, and indeed should be, therapeutic, just as our first glance at them or the sound of their voice on a telephone should be and is diagnostic.

A statement such as this is often challenged as reflecting an approach to practice of moving too quickly, jumping the gun, or responding to the client on the basis of our own biases, blind spots, and quick impressions. No doubt these risks exist. Thus an important component of this immediate diagnostic process is the high responsibility to be guarded, open, suspicious, and tentative about our judgments, to be cautious about moving too quickly but understanding the equally high risk of moving too slowly. In summary, we need to be aware that the judgment process is underway from the very beginning.

The acts of obtaining new information, processing it, assessing it, and judging its relevance need to be coterminous. It is this deliberation process, this function of discernment, that clearly separates our interaction with clients and their critical persons and environment from social interactions that are part of the day-to-day human interaction of our nonprofessional lives.

Often, to an untrained observer, the process of interviewing would appear to be no more nor less than a friendly, kindly interaction between two people in which one is probably doing much more listening than talking. What is not readily observable is the process of evaluation, critical thinking, and judging that is going on simultaneously and continuously. Indeed, often the more skilled a colleague becomes in therapeutic situations, the easier and less clinical the process appears. Unfortunately, it is because of this fact that the skill and knowledge required to interview effectively appear to be so uncomplicated that its difficulties and challenges tend to be discounted. "Surely any well-meaning person can sit and talk to people in a friendly way like that" is a comment that is still heard.

As the process of evaluating what the client is saying and not saying goes on, another process that we need to discern is the impact of the client on the worker and vice versa.

Most of these comments refer, of course, to that point of our practice, where we are in direct contact with clients. However, as social workers much of our practice in some settings involves interaction with others in the client's life, other systems, and other milieus. This work with significant others is not, as it once was, seen only as an information-gathering process but as part of evaluating the function as mentioned previously.

Over and over again, we are trying to determine four things:

1. Who are these clients as human persons?
2. What are their significant environments?
3. How do they interface and interact?
4. How can I or someone or something else be helpful to them?

This is, in essence, the combination of the history and assessment process out of which the diagnosis emerges.

An important part of this process of information gathering is to remind ourselves that the very decisions we make about what we need to know about a client are themselves a part of the combined assessment-diagnostic process. As already noted, we have thankfully moved well beyond that era in practice when we first thought we needed to know everything about a client and his or her life before we took action. Rather, throughout, the diagnostic and assessment process leads us to make the necessary decisions and judgments about relevance and significance.

Some of Mary Richmond's guidelines for material that are important in various situations are reflected in this earlier tendency to gather everything. (This influenced us for decades, even though she warned us that not everything in every one of her schedules was critical in every case.) We have learned well that often we need to know very little about clients and their lives in order to be helpful.

Apart from the unnecessary strain on clients and those we interview who are a part of their lives, our professional time is valuable and thus needs to be used sparingly and wisely, just as is the clients'. However, I think it is important to remind ourselves that in situations where we feel comfortable to proceed with a minimum base of knowledge that we have made a series of critical discerning judgments about the client's ability to function. That is, we have made a highly complex and sophisticated diagnosis.

But, as an aside, it is also important to remember that there may be many aspects of a client's life that we need not know about yet are important for the client to tell us. That is, the therapeutic gains in many interventions stem from the client's opportunity to be heard in an accepting, empathetic, supporting way. The information-sharing process in a therapeutic encounter goes two ways. On one hand, we must discover what we need to know in order to act responsibly, but on the other, we must learn what the client needs and wants to tell us in order to feel understood and be helped. Our diagnosis may lead us to judge that what is needed for the client is an opportunity to talk about himself or herself.

As we make decisions about what we want to know based on an ongoing series of judgments, unless we practice from some predetermined template, then each decision, as, for example, not to seek permission to talk to an adolescent's teacher, is a diagnostic one. Such a decision is beyond the assessment stage, for it says, "In my judgment, I do not need any more input from this area of the client's life." At times, of course, we do not know what a presenting situation is all about, and we will seek permission to extend our reach into the client's life beyond our face-to-face interviews. But such a decision is also an outcome of the diagnostic process. As was said earlier, one of the most important, succinct, and responsible diagnoses that we can make is to say, "I do not know what this is all about."

The diagnostic process is ongoing as we seek to discern the critical components that emerge from an assessment of a client and his or her reality, to which we need to be attentive as we seek to bring about with the client some type of change. Clearly, at times we will reorder our thinking, go back and clarify, seek the opinions of others, have the client help us, and have others help us to clarify our judgments.

Complicated and convoluted as this may sound, we need to remember that this whole process can take place in a very short time, the space of a ten-minute phone call or a fifteen-minute intake interview. So often these brief service contacts are seen not as service but as some type of administrative action. I have long thought that some of our most skilled diagnosticians and brief contact therapists are experienced intake workers who can deal effectively and helpfully with a broad range of presenting situations with minimum information in a single day.

I once participated in a research project that involved reaching out to persons who had been seen in what was then called an intake process but who did not come in for their first scheduled interview. This was during the time when the intake function was seen as administrative and partially diagnostic but certainly not therapeutic. Over and over again in our interviews with these persons, we were informed that they didn't come back because they had received the help they wanted at the intake interview. At first we viewed this as resistance and denial, according to the theory of the day. However, we soon learned that clients could quote chapter and verse describing their situations before they were seen and their present improved situations.

## The Record

But diagnosis also needs to be a fact. That is, in addition to addressing in a formal conscious way the ongoing process of diagnosis, there is also the responsibility to make a formal summary statement of it several times during a case. That is, somewhere there needs to be a written diagnosis, several times repeated, depending on the ongoing life of a case. (I include here in the term *written* the concept of a computer screen, a tape recording, etc., as forms of writing.)

It is here as a profession that we are weakest. That is why I argue so strongly that we must bring back the concept of diagnosis into our practice. Over and over again I have read case records with no indication of the social worker's judgments about the client. We need this recorded diagnosis for a variety of audiences: ourselves, the client, the agency, other social workers, other professions, and for our own profession.

As mentioned elsewhere, we have an ethical responsibility to diagnose. It is our public statement to those to whom we are accountable for our professional judgments to back up what we did or did not do in specific cases. If there is no tangible evidence of our diagnostic decisions, there is no way that we can be held accountable for the outcome of a case, except of course in those dramatic situations where persons are physically harmed or are highly dissatisfied with what has happened to them. Thankfully, many licensing and certification bodies now insist that proper records of cases be kept, and undoubtedly this will help ensure that some type of diagnostic material will be recorded.

But in addition to our more public responsibility, the advantage of a regularly formulated "written" diagnosis is that it assists us in the discipline of reviewing where we are, of identifying our levels of certainty and uncertainty, and if necessary to redirect our intervention with the client. This process of making periodic formal diagnostic statements reminds us of the warning given by Mary Richmond, many decades ago, about the imperfection and tentativeness of any and all diagnoses, a warning that needs to keep us humble and alert.

But we also diagnose for the client. That is, our diagnostic endeavors are to ensure a maximum level of precision and completeness to the process that in turn contributes greatly to ensure precision and thoroughness in treatment. As mentioned elsewhere, I am not saying that there is a direct relationship between diagnosis and a specific form of treatment that applies in all similar situations. That is, diagnosis A does not lead to a specific template of treatment B. What it does, however, is lead to a treatment that has a basis of rationality and thoroughness related to the diagnosis. When treatment is based on a strong and careful effort at diagnosis, there is a greater chance that it will be more effective than a more randomly selected strategy. Certainly, one can imagine that there are colleagues much more skilled in diagnosis than treatment; however, such situations should be rare if we view the diagnostic and treatment process as strongly intertwined.

When we speak of diagnosis as being for the client, an interesting aspect of current practice comes to mind. If we talk about diagnosing for the client, should or do clients have a right to know and see our diagnosis? Clearly, the tradition over the decades has been that records including diagnoses were a professional act from which the client was excluded even though virtually everyone else in an agency had access to them. Due to a variety of societal changes relative to disclosure and access to material concerning oneself, the rules, laws, and practices have changed so that now it is much more common for records, including diagnoses, to be accessible to clients and indeed to others in the client's life in particular situations.

An interesting question stemming from this new societal reality is whether the greater access and open records have had an impact on the "written diagnosis." That is, does the knowledge that our judgments about a client may be seen by the client and others in the client's life influence what we say about the client? I am certain that it does. As I look at records in various settings, although I have not done so in a systematic review process, I find a paucity of written diagnoses, indeed a paucity of what might be called assessments, except in a vague imprecise way that at times reflects the Kadushin (1963a) article "Diagnosis and Evaluation for (Almost) All Occasions." I do not know the answer to this conundrum. Responsible practice requires that we state clearly the basis on which we are taking professional action. Yet the current social climate strongly stresses that all of our decisions and documentation about clients are virtually an open book. What do we do about situations where we judge there is a risk of suicide, a possible risk to oneself, other workers, someone in the client's life or that a client is no longer able to function on his or her own, or that a marriage has little chance of succeeding? Clearly, we have to find some middle position. This is especially important when our concerns relate to high-risk situations and risks to ourselves, our clients, or others.

But we also diagnose for the setting or agency in which we function. Since everyone in a practice setting, including colleagues who are in private practice, need to know what is going on within a setting, it is necessary that the diagnostic process be recorded. That is, in each case the profile of diagnostic judgments made by practitioners needs to be available to those who have a right to it.

Although in practice we tend to view cases as our own, in most instances we are agents of some administrative structure and in reality our clients are also clients of the setting. This becomes clear in litigious situations where suit is brought against not only the individual therapist but also the agency as a whole. I am not sure that this is as obvious in situations where groups of colleagues are practicing privately in some loose collegial arrangement. It certainly needs to be considered.

But also, we must have formal diagnoses for others who may need to have access to our records when we are not present to speak of a case, or in emergencies or situations where a case is being transferred either within the agency or to another service or profession. Here I believe our responsibility to have available clear and concise diagnoses is imperative for several reasons. The first is to ensure that a client is not required to go through a long process of exploration, negotiation, and clarification. Clients have often told me that they had to tell their story several times as they moved through the referral process in order to find the most appropriate kind and source of help.

We need to record diagnoses to give our colleagues a running start on a case, both to save time and, more important, to give the client a continuity as far as possible. Of course, our colleagues have a responsibility to formulate their own diagnoses and will use our own as only one component of it.

We also have a responsibility to diagnose to protect our colleagues. This is an area where I have great concern. I am thinking of situations where we believe a person to have a high suicide risk, or to be a danger to professionals, or to have a high probability of harming others, such as a partner or children, but do not record this because we believe we should not categorize or label people in this way. I suggest that it is seriously unethical to not identify clearly in our records judgments we have made about such risk situations so that any colleague who comes later will be alerted. Obviously, in making these judgments we face the risk of being wrong, but the reverse is too dangerous to even consider. In such situations, as mentioned elsewhere, we need to record our degree of certainty about such a judgment.

We also have a responsibility to record diagnoses for the profession in general. In a profession as broadly focused and dynamic as social work, indeed in any profession, we need to be committed to an ongoing process of knowledge building. Clearly, there are many ways in which knowledge emerges or develops. A principle way in our discipline is a constant process of evaluating what we do, to whom we do it, when we do it, and with what outcomes. Over and over again, recent research has shown that from an overall perspective, regardless of setting or theoretical orientation, what we do with clients is effective in bringing about a level and kind of change with which they are satisfied. The great challenge we now face is to move from this general knowledge of effectiveness to a much more precise one. We must learn more about whom we help, in what circumstances, and under what conditions; of course, implied here is the equally important question of whom do we not help and whom we only help a little, but not as much as we would like. We can address this in many ways, but surely one of the most important is to obtain much more data than we presently have on the correlation between diagnosis, intervention, and outcome. Is there a direct relationship among these three factors, or is outcome a much more idiosyncratic result of the person and his or her relationships?

However, even if future research indicated that our diagnosis of a client and the outcome of the helping process are not clearly interconnected, this in no way would diminish our responsibility to diagnose clearly and accurately. We have learned both individually and as a profession over the decades just how powerful the relationship between a client and a professional can be. Unfortunately, we know all too well that this power can also cause harm, indeed serious harm when it is misunderstood by either the social worker or the client, or even worse when it is deliberately abused by the practitioner. Again, we will only understand such situations accurately when we are in a position to review professional opinions or judgments that the worker has made which led to the relationship becoming a medium of hurt rather than help.

Written diagnoses should be available to the public when this is appropriate. In a general way, the public presumes that professionals in a discipline such as ours are held accountable by various public bodies, such as legislative bodies or colleges or boards. In recent years these bodies have increasingly included members from outside the particular discipline as well as making their procedures public to some extent.

A part of this process of public accountability is the understanding that a professional person needs to function from a discipline-based body of knowledge and account for what is done or not done in particular cases on the basis of an appropriate judgment of the essential features of a case. The fact that increasing numbers of cases involving social workers are being examined either in the open arena of the public press, in the more formal structure of professional discipline committees, or just as frequently in court, causes considerable discomfort to many in the profession.

What does not seem to be understood is that this development is a strong positive recognition of the profession and of the importance and desirability of quality, accountable social work services. Two separate but connected themes seem to mark these cases. The first asks whether the social worker acted appropriately with the client. This type of situation reflects issues of professional conduct in a general sense. The other type of case, which appears to be increasing in frequency, relates to the topic of diagnosis. Did the worker make a correct series of judgments about the situation based on the knowledge available? Did the worker make a correct diagnosis? In other words, would an equally qualified practitioner have been expected to make the critical judgments in regard to what was done or not done in the case? In recent years in many countries, cases such as this involve questions of risk to children. In many instances, the available records do not adequately indicate what judgments were made about a situation except through inference in relation to actions that were taken. In such cases, practitioners are rightly criticized for a failure to be explicit in recording their diagnoses. But in all instances, society expects a professional person to keep appropriate records that show the basis on which action was taken, that is, that a diagnosis was made.

In summary, this chapter has emphasized and attempted to show the importance of seeing diagnosis both as a process and a record. Neither side of this duality is of greater importance than the other. Both are essential. The trap of seeing diagnosis in a unitary sense was underlined and the need to understand both what diagnosis means and does not mean was underscored.

# Chapter 10

# Diagnosis and Gut Reaction

A term that for a long time I found distasteful and conceptually troubling is *gut reaction*. I presume that it is of North American origin as I have not heard it, nor seen it used, in other countries. I first began to hear this term from recent graduates about fifteen years ago. Quite often in encountering new colleagues I would politely ask them how they were getting on in their respective practices. Frequently they would tell me that early in their new positions they had been advised by so-called seasoned co-workers, "Now that you are out of school you can forget all that theory and diagnostic stuff and get on with some real social work practice in which one does best by following one's gut reaction."

This idea of the key to effective intervention appears to mean that one ought to avoid a cognitive approach to practice but rather should follow one's visceral responses to, and instincts about, a case. Clearly, this concept of practice was not and is not widespread, but I have heard of it and I am sure others have as well, sufficiently often to make it a matter that I believe should be addressed.

Apart from the inelegance of the term and its clearly nonprofessional origins, this idea of spontaneity rather than a more logical and planned approach to practice seems to contradict entirely our century-old struggle to understand the process of social work treatment to make it more effective. At first I was irritated at colleagues who espoused this concept and handed it on to new social workers as "real social work." I presumed they had abandoned a commitment to responsible practice. However, I was also puzzled by it, for I knew that persons of this disposition saw themselves and were seen as effective, responsible practitioners. As I thought more about it, I concluded that this thinking mode stemmed from the perception that diagnosis was coidentified with the assignment of labels by practitioners through a rational process that excluded the client.

My negative reaction to this position began to change following an experience a few years ago when a senior colleague and I, appearing on a panel, were asked to comment on a case summary with which we were presented. I discussed the case from several theoretical perspectives and in a diagnostic framework that led me to some suggestions for possible treatment goals. My colleague, someone whom I well respected, politely began his commentary by saying that he believed in neither theory nor diagnosis. He went on to say that over the years he had learned in his practice how to "tune in to a client and follow his or her responses to the visceral cues" he experienced. (I don't recall that he actually said "gut.")

However, what fascinated me about his discussion of the case was his rich understanding of it, an ability to see subtleties of person and situation and to convey a most empathetic and sensitive response to the material. What struck me then, and as I thought about it later, was the diagnostic acumen this colleague demonstrated, a skill in picking up and putting together the essential details of where the client was, as seen in the record. Also, I admired the imaginative way he suggested of working with the client based on this demonstrated ability to cut quickly to the core of the situation. As I heard him speak, I realized that he was a highly skilled colleague who clearly would be helpful to the persons with whom he had professional contact. In summary, in spite of his protestations to the contrary, in my eyes at least, this colleague knew a great deal of theory and applied it in a highly sensitive diagnostic manner, but in a manner that appeared to be totally intuitive and spontaneous.

Since then I have altered my former negative views on this way of describing practice and I pay much more attention to it. I do so because I believe that we have much to learn from our skilled colleagues who make rich diagnoses very quickly, accurately, and apparently without thought but rather by confidence in their emotive responses to a client. Unfortunately, as we have done so frequently in our history, we have made an incorrect dichotomy between persons who apparently act principally in a spontaneous manner and those whose practice reflects a more cerebral process, presuming that one was right and one was wrong. The unfortunate aspect of this division is that it is cast as the diagnosticians versus the nondiagnosticians, or the theorists versus the practitioners—another example of the old diagnostic-functional schism. It also reflects the split between rationality and emotion or empathy.

Having pondered this for some time, I challenge this dichotomy. I am now convinced that we can best see this phenomenon as a continuum rather than a dichotomy. Remember what Helen Perlman told us, that regardless of our stated views on diagnosis we indeed all diagnose. Clearly some of us do so almost automatically as we become more skilled and experienced, and others do so in a more overtly cognitive manner.

Over and over again, I am impressed with the level of sensitivity and accuracy that many colleagues show in describing clients, yet I am disappointed and worried that in so many instances, regardless of their view of practice, they have not followed through in their records with the formulation of a diagnosis. The issue seems to hinge on our perception of diagnosis or perhaps our misperceptions about it. Nevertheless, I stand convinced that these so-called antidiagnosticians are in fact highly skilled, perceptive, and accurate diagnosticians.

If indeed such colleagues are skilled diagnosticians, they are of course not the only ones who are. I think it would be tragic if these colleagues who follow their "gut reactions" were held up as the models of practice to be emulated by neophyte social workers. I raise this issue lest we suggest that persons who are committed to the discipline of careful assessments and specified diagnoses can be viewed as lacking empathy. I also worry that a perception could develop that our spontaneous emotive responses, by definition, are always accurate, helpful, and therapeutic and cognition is not. These two qualities can, and indeed must, exist together in practitioners.

I am suggesting that there is much to be learned from those who are known to be quality practitioners even though they purport to practice from a nontheory, nondiagnostic base. Our task is to find better processes of learning about the judgments they make in what appears to be a nonconceptual process that leads them to move in particular directions with clients. Clearly the mission of this volume is that not only should we learn from them, but we should find ways of helping such colleagues to translate their observable skill in the process of diagnosis into an equal skill in the description and recording of diagnosis.

Certainly, as one speculates on this phenomenon of responding to clients in an apparently noncognitive style, the skill developed in meditation comes to mind. To an increasing extent, social workers are turning to the various schools of meditation as a way of both developing self-enlightenment and helping clients for whom such practices are appropriate to make use of the potential of meditation for self-growth. Many social workers who have learned to meditate report that as their meditation skill develops, so too do their attending abilities. These abilities in turn facilitate their ability to connect to a broader range of people more quickly and more intensively in a nonrational noncognitive way. These attending skills are not to be discounted. There is growing evidence of the improved communication skills that develop as a secondary gain in the process of learning to meditate (Keefe).

But as those who have engaged in the discipline of learning to meditate know, considerable self-discipline and practice are required. Interestingly, the goal of meditation is to learn to experience life and all aspects of ourselves in a nonrational manner. This skill seems to be similar to the skill of practitioners who experience a client's situation without consciously using a cognitive process. By using the same discipline as a tool in learning how to meditate, our responsibility, both to the profession and ourselves, is an attempt to explain in a cognitive, replicable way, our understanding of a client and the source and credibility of this understanding.

If indeed it is a worthwhile goal to attempt to alter the attitude and practice of some aspects of the profession's mores, it would seem important that we attempt to understand the behaviors we are trying to influence. As I have thought more about the view that we should "only trust our impressions," in particular their sources in our professional ethos, several ideas have come to mind.

Certainly, from an ideological perspective there is a flavor of postmodern thinking in this approach to practice, a body of thought which urges that we turn away from an overly scientific approach to practice toward a much more experiential one. The postmodern stance urges us to be more holistic in our practice and open to new ideas and understandings of the human condition, whatever their source.

I think that we can understand the antipathy to the concept of diagnosis from the perspective of some of the issues discussed in Chapter 2. Certainly, the idea that diagnosis is related to the first judgments we make about people on meeting them has rarely been highlighted in our literature. Rather, especially in earlier decades, diagnosis was seen as a very formal, time-bound, intellectual exercise that follows the process of social history or social assessment. Even though throughout our history our literature has said that the process of diagnosis begins in our first contact with a client, we have not done a good job of transmitting this idea to the profession in general.

Neither have we been overly successful in communicating the concept of diagnosis as both a process and a record. In stressing the recording of diagnosis, we have minimized the more essential aspect of the process. We have also greatly minimized the complexity of the process, especially overlooking that the essence of this process is the ongoing series of judgments we make in any human interaction, be it social or professional. I suspect that historically we have been so committed to the position that we cannot be judgmental in our interactions with clients that we find it difficult to learn that this is very different from making judgments about them.

Further, as discussed earlier, the word *diagnosis* itself has been given a pejorative meaning in much of the academic social work literature, and thus for some the politically correct position is to be against diagnosis. With this mind-set it is understandable that diagnosis is frequently not observable in our practice.

Finally and perhaps most seriously, to date, as a profession, we have not made a strong case that underscores the importance, indeed even the necessity of a social diagnosis. We know that many clients are helped through the process of having an opportunity to be heard, accepted, and understood by a concerned, knowledgeable professional. We know also that many clients are in fact competent, healthy, and well-functioning but need, or perceive that they need, assistance with some aspect of their lives. Thus, in many instances our diagnostic process may be quite incorrect and still cause little harm. However, because we also see the very multifaceted damaged people of the world in life and death situations in which a mistake can be tragic, indeed fatal, it is necessary that we always diagnose both in process and in writing.

One of the many serious outcomes of an approach to practice that ignores or minimizes a commitment to diagnosis is that it greatly impedes our ongoing responsibility to study the different impact of our interventions. Both from our internal acceptance of responsibility for what we do, and an increasing societal demand for accountability, the next two decades are going to be marked by a strong demand to demonstrate the outcomes of our interventions.

We need to demonstrate not only what happens when we engage in particular strategies with clients but why it happens. To be accountable, it is essential that we set out in a clear and consistent way our understanding of each professional situation and how this understanding leads us to take whatever intervention steps occur.

As we move in this direction, let us hope that more and more of our highly competent clinicians will subject themselves to the discipline of recording their diagnoses so that we learn from them. I, for one, will attempt to stop seeing them as irresponsible and deficient in their practice but rather set my sights on finding ways to tap their diagnostic competence in a manner by which all can benefit. Indeed, I think I can live comfortably with their definition of their diagnostic skill as "gut reaction" as long as they commit themselves to summarize the reactions on which they base their interventions with the individuals, couples, groups, and families whom they serve.

# Chapter 11

# Diagnosis and Assessment

Throughout the process of writing the previous chapters I have been haunted by a question: Has anything been said thus far about diagnosis and its meaning that does not apply to the term *assessment,* which appears to have replaced, or rather substituted for, diagnosis in much of the social work literature, especially in North America? If the answer is no, then why try to undo something that seems to be comfortably entrenched in our practice lore?

It is my thesis that the answer is yes. This shift in terminology is more than a substitution of words. Rather, I believe it to be a misguided effort to change an integral and long-standing conceptual base of practice, to the detriment of the clients.

Of course it is easy to assert this gratuitously. But I must proffer reasons for stating this position. I view the challenge as twofold: I must first consider whether in fact there is a difference between the concepts of diagnosis and assessment. If so, both terms should be used with their own proper meaning. Second, and more difficult to address, is whether what we are looking at in practice is really only a word substitution and that conceptually both mean the same thing.

It is the thesis of this book that there is an important difference between diagnosis and assessment. Both are important. Both are needed in the profession's lexicon to help bring further precision to our practice and our understanding of practice. Both can aid us in better serving our clients. By attempting to substitute one for the other, we lose an important focusing concept and diminish the precision we need.

As the book's title suggests, even though diagnosis is a term that has been misused, it is an essential term to which we should give more precision. Thus, rather than ban it from the shelves of our accumulated wisdom, it should be returned from its exile and reinstated to its former position of eminence. I am not suggesting that this is a question of right or wrong; I see it rather as a matter of strategy that has import for our clients, which is hopefully what we are all about.

I am certain that many of our conceptualizers of practice, with the best of intentions, have chosen to substitute assessment for diagnosis because of the supposed failings and clear misuses of the term *diagnosis* with no intention of modifying our responsibility to conceptually based practice. That is, they take the position that the two terms are synonymous, with one being preferred to the other. If one looks at the definition of assessment in the most recent edition of Barker's (1991) *Social Work Dictionary*, it comes close to the concept of diagnosis as used here, apart from the emphasis on problem that it contains. Nevertheless, I suggest strongly that, in fact, diagnosis is the preferred term and should be the one we use.

I have identified six reasons why I believe both terms are needed in today's practice world:

1. Diagnosis is still an acceptable and precious term within the profession.
2. Assessment and diagnosis are different.
3. The usage of assessment only appears to result in less rigor in recording.
4. The sociopolitics of professions demand it.
5. Clients pay a price for this kind of word substitution.
6. The profession pays a price as well.

### Diagnosis Is Still an Acceptable and Precious Term Within the Profession

I began writing this book from a somewhat presumptuous self-assumed "voice from the wilderness" stance. I did this out of a conviction and concern that the term *diagnosis* had virtually disappeared from the professional literature of social work. To come to this conclusion I had used several sources. I first conducted a review of the current textbooks on social work practice most frequently used in schools and faculties of social work. Second, I drew upon the comments about diagnosis found in the various editions of *The Social Work Dictionary* and the most recent editions of the *Encyclopedia of Social Work* published by the National Association of Social Workers. Last, I was urged by the tenor of many discussions with other academics, most of whom viewed me as being out of step.

In these venues I have experienced a haughty dismissal of the term in a less than friendly manner, based on the simplistic arguments either that diagnosis referred to pathology and thus should be eschewed, or more commonly by dragging out our oft-used scapegoat, the famous so-called medical model. And of course all social workers know that we do not like "the medical model," if indeed such a singular model exists!

But in spite of its rejection in much of our textbook literature, even there it is important to note some exceptions. Principally I refer to the five editions of the preeminent volume by Hollis, then Woods. Here there has been a consistency in maintaining the term *diagnosis* albeit with some accommodation to the trend toward assessment. As well, to date the four very successful editions of *Differential Diagnosis and Treatment in Social Work* (Turner, 1995) have been consistent in this regard.

However, as I continued the literature search beyond the course books, I found that the term was used much more in our practice journals than I would have expected. That is, as discussed in Chapter 2, a significant group of practitioners, particularly in the micro practice field, continue to use the term in a traditional "taken for granted," way. I have not examined fully this apparent dichotomy, but as speculated in Chapter 2, this dichotomy of usage may be another example of the long-standing town-gown division that has manifested in the sociology of other professions.

Last, when I examined the legislation for social work in various jurisdictions, I found that the word *diagnosis* appeared in more than a few definitions of practice. Thus my quest is not to reinstate diagnosis as I first thought but to restore it to its previous place of eminence.

### Assessment and Diagnosis Are Different

In my view, the most important reason for not abandoning diagnosis for assessment is because the two concepts, although closely allied, are distinct and describe two different facets of the intervention process. Thus, by attempting to combine their separate meanings into a single term, we lose some of the richness and, more important, the preciseness of each.

As the concept has emerged over the profession's history, assessment has referred to that process of looking at the broad sweep of a client's life and reality as it emerges throughout the life of the case, deciding on the importance or lack thereof, and assessing its specific relevance for the emerging picture. This is particularly important for social work because of the broad spectrum of potentially critical aspects of a client's life that we know may significantly influence his or her psychosocial reality of today.

Assessment, like diagnosis, is going on all the time. However, in assessment we are trying to ascertain which parts of a client's life are critical and essential to understanding the client's goals and aspirations for the treatment process. An important quality of assessment is to save the client, and us, from gathering, reviewing, and analyzing large amounts of information, as once was our style in the days of preparing detailed and thorough social histories.

In assessment, we are continually letting our searchlights, using a variety of theoretical lenses, sweep the client's person, life, and reality to watch for areas that appear to be significant for the case. It is the process that flags important areas of strength and present stress. It is not trying to tie these all together but rather attempting to get a reading on the client's overall person-in-situation and breaking out the critical areas for attention in the treatment process.

Diagnosis takes this process further. The task of diagnosis is to look at our conclusions in the assessment phase as to what is important and to begin to analyze and judge how they fit together, to give us a picture of what is essential to know in order to proceed planfully with this situation. In some ways, assessment can be seen as the roving searchlight that scans the large picture and diagnosis as the microscope that give us precision and focus.

Clearly, these are not sequential activities. Assessment is a much more disciplined and individualized concept than was the earlier process of study or history taking allegedly followed by diagnosis. There is, of course, a judgment factor in assessment, an important component of which relates to a respect for and commitment to parsimony. Hence, assessment seeks to avoid fishing expeditions that attempt to gather all that is knowable about the client before any action is taken. Assessment is a process that leads us to quickly drop a topic when it is clear that it is of little importance either for the worker or the client.

Diagnosis, then, functions as the process of taking the pieces emerging as significant and seeking to put them together in a manner that reflects where in our judgment the client is in a manner that gives us sufficient security to act or not. Clearly, it would be wrong to overstress the differences between these two processes, just as I believe we have greatly understressed the differences that do exist to minimize the supposed rigidity and overrationalization in diagnosis. One could visualize these two processes as a constant back and forth motion, in which assessment finds something interesting and diagnosis pursues further to see if it is relevant or not.

### The Usage of Assessment Only Appears to Result in Less Rigor in Recording

As I continue to examine the way assessment is commonly used in the literature, I believe that this usage tends to result in a process that is less rigorous than diagnosis. This may be unfair to the authors who favor assessment over diagnosis and who stress as strongly as I would our ongoing responsibility to know what we are doing in practice. However, I sense that for many assessment conveys a less rigorous approach to the process of conscious formulation of judgments on which to base intervention.

This assertion stems from my observations in practice. As I have examined agency records over the last decade, I have noticed a greatly diminished presence of what might be called a diagnosis or diagnostic summary, whether this is called assessment or not, that is, a statement modified through the life of the case as to who the client is judged to be, the nature of service being given, and the basis on which we decide to act in particular ways.

What I do observe with admiration is the richness and depth of our knowledge and understanding of clients as I look at case outcomes. These outcomes demonstrate our ability to connect to clients, to hear them, and with them to sort out the areas of life where they are hurting and/or where their strengths lie.

However, often the section of the record that is called assessment is only a summary of historical material given by the client. What is so often lacking is information as to how the practitioner decided to proceed in a particular direction. I frequently ask myself, Does this colleague realize how much he or she has helped this client or family or group? Does this colleague realize how dangerous this person is? Does this colleague realize that this mother is asking for help for herself, not her partner?

The point is that seeing assessment as a substitute for our former commitment to diagnose, even if we misunderstood the proper parameters of a social work diagnosis, can lead to an avoidance of our responsibility to state loudly and clearly in our records on what basis have we decided to take or not take professional action. This is the true purpose of diagnosis.

## The Sociopolitics of Professions Demand It

My fourth reason to urge the reinstatement of diagnosis along with, not instead of, assessment stems from a sociopolitical perspective. In our society, and most particularly among the professions with whom we interact, diagnosis is an accepted, highly respected, and essential function. It is much broader than a search for pathology or problem. It is presumed that responsible, ethical practitioners, whatever their discipline, need to diagnose. Members of other professions seriously question a profession such as ours which at times proudly proclaims that it does not diagnose. We seem to be the last profession that wants to let other professions own the term.

Yes, of course, physicians diagnose, but they do medical diagnoses. The same is true of a broad range of other disciplines and professions, such as veterinarians, psychologists, teachers, dietitians, and others. In each instance, professions insist that they do only diagnoses appropriate to their discipline. We may not like how some professions interpret the process themselves, but in no way should that affect our application of the concept.

Hence, social workers do only social work diagnoses, and when we do so we are not mimicking other professions. What we are doing is acting in a manner demanded of any professional. At times components of our diagnosis will overlap with a diagnosis made by a colleague on another person. So be it! There are many overlapping concepts and activities among all professions. At times there are and should be commonalties in the way a particular situation is judged. This is to be encouraged, applauded, and expected as we move to more permeable boundaries between the helping professions.

In each instance when a professional diagnosis has been made, the one diagnosing has to be prepared to take responsibility. I recently read a case report where the worker correctly judged and stated that the client was "very depressed" yet took no action, to the serious detriment of the client.

There are several ways in which opting out of a responsibility to diagnose can affect us. When we publicly declare that we do not diagnose, we can be excluded from various kinds of legislation that could be tremendously important to our clients; our clients can lose access to some types of insurance that require a diagnosis, and we can lose our clients' respect for us. Clients expect us to "social work them" and to feed back to them our opinions about them and their situations.

Many other groups in society are comfortable with their responsibility to diagnose as a highly respected part of their armamentarium of skills. Hence, my auto mechanic lists diagnostic services as one of his functions, as does my daughter's cosmetician. Just a few weeks ago I received an advertisement from a well-known telephone company offering to come to the house to diagnose my telephone requirements.

In summary, I am suggesting that our seeming reluctance to use the terminology of diagnosis out of a misguided fear that we would be mimicking another profession represents much more discomfort with responsibility than any quality of immaturity. The immaturity, if any, lies in our fear of responsibility and of being wrong.

## Clients Pay a Price for This Kind of Word Substitution

The next argument in support of the use of diagnosis as well as assessment relates to the well-being of our clients. One of the principle reasons I am addressing this topic is a growing realization that our reluctance to use the term *diagnosis* and our denial that it is a proper function of social work results in clients being deprived of service in at least three different ways.

In a bureaucratic way, failure to diagnose can result in clients being unable to access various forms of insurance benefits or health schemes that require a diagnosis before services will be covered. This is a complex matter, for such programs themselves often have an oversimplified concept of diagnosis by code that requires a highly restricted categorization of problem and service—a concept of diagnosis that we all rightly resist. However, I suggest that in the long run it is better for the clients if we wage this struggle in terms of demanding a broader understanding of social work diagnosis rather than proclaiming that we do not diagnose.

A second way in which clients can suffer from a lack of diagnostic commitment is to deprive them of access to existing services. For example, if services exist to treat such things as attention deficit disorders, phobias, or eating disorders, etc., and we take a position that we do not use such labels or classifications in our assessments and thus certainly would never diagnose such disorders, then how can our clients make use of these resources? We can, of course, avoid responsibility by a referral strategy that avoids making a diagnosis and lets others do it for us. This frequently results in clients unnecessarily having to go through an assessment and diagnostic process that we could and should have carried out.

Well-formulated diagnoses can greatly enhance the possibility of our clients being accepted for services by other settings. It is in my view unethical to put clients in situations where they have to undergo a vigorous diagnostic process that would not have taken place if we had already done it, having had sufficient contact with, and understanding of, the client to do so.

A third way in which clients can suffer from a lack of diagnostic commitment occurs when, because of the lack of precision and discipline required in a diagnosis, we fail to recognize that a particular action, resource, or help is needed. This is of particular concern in relation to colleagues who seem to pride themselves on their ability to intuit who and where a client is. That is, the process of assessment leading toward diagnosis is viewed as an emotion-based response, not a logical, reasoned one where alternatives are considered and conscious judgments are formulated.

A particular area of concern is well-masked depression and suicidal intent that are not always conveyed through emotional messages and nonverbal cues. As discussed in another section, the critical role of intuition and visceral response to a client is not being discounted as a source of information. What is being challenged is making this the sole basis on which treatment decisions are made.

### The Profession Pays a Price As Well

A further way in which letting assessment stand for or replace diagnosis is harmful is that the profession suffers. Although of course there is a self-serving aspect in looking after professional interests, in the long run, it is the clients and the public who pay the price.

Because diagnosis is so powerful and indeed dangerous, yet necessary, it is considered very precious to the helping professions in general. Some legislation even designates which professions are authorized to diagnose in a manner appropriate to them. Just as being recognized as a senior profession, a position that we have long held, is important, so too is the vocabulary that accompanies this status.

Professional vocabulary is a part of the power structure of a profession. Without this power we cannot empower clients or help them to empower themselves from the strengths of our position. To declare that social work is not among the senior helping professions because we are uncomfortable about the responsibility and risks inherent in such membership by failing to diagnose weakens our position within the cadre of professions. We also do this by hiding our diagnostic processes in what appears to be a softer, less risky word. In both these instances, our ability to influence significant power structures in a client's life is also weakened.

In recent years in my own province there have been several situations where social work was excluded from a list of professions eligible to perform particular functions because of an earlier position that we do not diagnose. (This situation has been rectified in recent scope of practice statements adopted by the professional association.)

An unfortunate and indeed embarrassing situation arises when some type of eligibility request needs to be signed off based on the formulation of a diagnosis by a psychologist, for example, because members of the profession are unwilling to diagnose.

As mentioned earlier, it is not the whole profession who has taken this position. However, a sufficiently large segment of highly visible and influential members of the profession, such as the authors of some of our well-known textbooks take a negative position on this matter. This position has tremendous influence on the upcoming generation of colleagues, as I have experienced in many dialogues with students who strongly wish to use politically correct terminology.

In summary, my position is that we should avoid any further efforts at declaring that we assess rather than diagnose and strive to return to a position which recognizes the subtle but critical difference between these two processes and ensures that both are a part of the lexicon of our practice and conceptual worlds.

# Chapter 12

# Diagnosis and Theory

One of the distinguishing attributes of contemporary social work practice is the richness of our theoretical base because of the plurality of theories. Although there would probably be some differences in opinion on just how many different theories or models of social work practice there are, we could presume there are more than twenty-five, with several others emerging. How this plurality relates to diagnosis is an intriguing and important question.

There are many ways to differentiate theories from one another. An important one is the use of particular vocabulary proper to the theory to describe various facets of intervention. This has at least three components. First, some theories use terminology common to other theories but give these common concepts a unique meaning. Other theories introduce new terminology to describe concepts that are viewed similarly across some or all theoretical lines. For example, existential theory prefers the label *encounter* rather than *relationship,* although its concept of relationship is similar to that in many other theories. Last, other theories introduce new terminology to describe new phenomena. Systems theory, for example, has introduced new concepts and new vocabulary. Some of its terminology has now become a part of the general lexicon of the profession.

The concept of diagnosis and how it is labeled is an important case in point. It touches on two of the above phenomena. All theories assume that social work practice must be based on some form of accountability, which implies that the worker knows what he or she is doing and is prepared to be responsible for it. There is a presumption of some type of diagnostic activity, although it may not be designated as such.

For many of the reasons discussed earlier, in some theories the word *diagnosis* is avoided and *assessment* is much preferred, seeming to imply that these two concepts are coterminous in social work. Hence, in comparing theories it is important to examine not only the preferred terminology in a theory but what is meant by it. For example, for some theories, although assessment is the preferred term, the concept includes what has been described in these pages as diagnosis. Thus, when discussions or presentations indicate that a particular theory does not use diagnosis, it is critical that we examine what is meant by this, as it may well be diagnosis by another name.

The other way in which theories vary is in the use of the term itself. Several current social work theories do use the term *diagnosis* but have different perceptions about what it means. For example, both ego psychology and existential theory include diagnosis in their purview of intervention but differ on what is meant by the term. Last, in other theories, neither assessment nor diagnosis is used, yet the concept of responsibility based on a set of judgments is present and stressed.

A further reason why the interface between diagnosis and theory needs to be given more attention relates to an important development in social work practice. This is the growing interest in, awareness of, and commitment to the necessity of practicing from a pluralistic theory base. Although there was once a search for a unitary theoretical base for practice, we now know that multiple theories are needed. Our practice is now so complex and the range of factors that influence clients so broad that no one theory can explain our total professional purview. No theory is better than another. Each has something to contribute.

As we better understand that each theory brings a new perspective on some aspect of our clients' lives and our practice, we can begin to view theories as resources that are to be used differently according to the client, the situation, and the setting in which we meet. Indeed, a very useful practice in situations of uncertainty is to formulate a diagnosis from two or three theoretical perspectives.

We have come far from a position that theory belongs to the practitioner, not the client or the setting. Such a viewpoint presumes that each of us develops our own theoretical base upon which our purview of practice is built. Rather, in social work theories are currently viewed as tools or resources of treatment that can be differentially applied. As we begin to view theories in this way and as we become more skillful in using different approaches to fit who and where the client is and wants to be rather than what we would prefer, we begin to understand how some theories fit better than others.

For example, we know different theories have differing value bases about the world, our relationship to it, and the goals and objectives that motivate us. Our clients also have different value bases, and thus some theories will be more congruent with a client than others.

Since different theories have different impacts, it follows that just as some theories are better suited for particular clients than others, it is likely that some theories can be harmful and upsetting to clients even though they may be congruent with a view of practice and the world with which we are highly identified.

This question of the differential use of theory has been discussed elsewhere (Turner 1996). It is raised here to introduce the concept that an important part of the judgment process needs to be a consideration of the overall value set of the client from his or her own perspective. Then a decision needs to be taken as to what strategy of intervention is indicated related to that value set. That is, which theories appear to best suit this client.

As basic a thing as a client's time orientation is an example of this point. Thus, some of our theories stress understanding, and helping the client understand, that what is happening now is related to his or her history. Other theories are much more future oriented and aim at helping the client overlook the past, start from the present, and move forward. If our theoretical orientation stresses the past and the client is much more forward looking or vice versa, a stressful situation could occur in treatment that could negate any possibility of a helpful process. Such differences are often very subtle and can easily be interpreted by us as blocking or resistance in clients, or perhaps a lack of motivation, when in fact it reflects a difference in perspective between practitioner and client.

Another component of the theory-diagnosis relationship is the methodology we choose to use in particular situations. This too is partially related to our theoretical base. Again, a client's view of the world and how problems are best worked on may be very group oriented while ours may be much more individualistically focused, or vice versa. Failing to appreciate this value difference could radically affect the process. The critical point here is that, as we have long known, our theoretical orientations influence how we view the world and the process of helping. When our worldviews are congruent with those of the client, then the possibility of a productive goodness of fit with the client is enhanced. Otherwise, the therapeutic situation can be stress producing and indeed harmful. Thus, regardless of the terminology used to describe the process, an important component of diagnosis is to address the client's overall value base.

One of the assumptions here is that, different as each theory may appear to be, each addresses the same spectrum of variables. If this is so, then there may be more similarity in the content and process of diagnosis than is usually imagined. Thus, although the essential structure of each diagnosis would have much in common, the emphasis, content, and vocabulary of it would vary from the perspective of different theories. That is, if indeed we are all concerned about the same variables in our clients' lives, then our theories will attempt to address the same spectrum of items or questions and differ only in the emphasis and importance they are given. The same idea applies to diagnosis. The work of Rachelle Dorfman (1988) in having a group of practitioners from different theoretical backgrounds review and comment on the same case demonstrated the extent of similarity in how cases were viewed. The differences related more to what was to be done and how, rather than who the clients were.

However, as one examines the range of thirty-some theories currently of some significance in contemporary social work practice, one variable on which they differ is the very concept of diagnosis and the use of the term. Since for some the term conveys only a search for pathology it is abhorred; for others, it is a one-time labeling of a client and thus is rejected; and so on. Thus, trying to establish how colleagues from different orientations view this process is somewhat daunting, not only because of conceptual differences in the theory but because of the vocabulary of each system and the meaning attributed to various concepts. Thus, if diagnosis is viewed in a narrow pathology-oriented manner and hence eschewed, then the task of identifying the process of judgment formation is made difficult by this barrier of terminology.

Nevertheless, if there is a common core of meaning to the process of assuming responsibility for our actions, then we must address the challenge of understanding different terminology. Clearly, as a beginning we can agree that we all work from a commitment to understand the person-in-situation equation with which we are faced.

Using any theory, a practitioner wants to know about the clients, their strengths, their aspirations, and their views of the world and of the helping process. Each theory accounts for the kinds, sources, and manifestation of stress and hurt, although these might be valued differently . Differentially, each theory requires examination of the client's immediate life situation, its strengths and limitations. Each prompts us to learn if the client is hurting and how, where, and why. Each sees the helping relationship as important although in a different perspective. Each involves a sense of time, basic human nature, and basic patterning of interrelationships. Each views accountability as essential, and each views itself as dynamic and open, although persons using some theoretical orientations may challenge the degree of openness claimed by others.

In no way is it being suggested that in fact we are moving toward any form of unified theory. Indeed, the reverse is true. I am only suggesting that each of our theories attempts to come to terms with a similar profile of variables. The reason it is exciting for the profession is that there are vast differences in how each theory deals with these variables. The advantage, as we move toward a worldwide multicultural practice, is that we have available to us a broad range of conceptual responses, which permits us in turn to respond to a broad range of worldviews and differences among persons.

Although much of this is as yet speculative, it appears to be worthwhile to pursue. One way that this might be done is to first see if indeed there is consensus among adherents to each of our current theories on what are the essential judgment calls, regardless of what we call the process. If so, this same coterie of colleagues could examine a case history from the perspective of what is judged to be essential, encouraging each to use whatever vocabulary or terminology he or she wishes.

As we move in this direction, we should be very careful to avoid standardizing the content or format of our diagnoses. Rather, I think we should foster diversity and see what we could learn from it rather than push for a uniformity that may only be reached by forcing data and concepts.

Although it is not my hope nor wish that we reach conceptual uniformity, we must do more in examining and identifying where we do agree in concept if not in terminology. Although such activities could be yet another interesting academic exploration, what is of critical importance is the client. For if we accept that we can harm clients by misusing theories or with misdiagnosis, then we have a strong ethical responsibility to give much more attention to the interface of theory, diagnosis, intervention, and outcome.

In so doing, we can better determine who we help, when, how, and from what perspective as well as who we hurt, when, and how in the complex realities of our practices. Our commitment as a profession, strengthened by over a hundred years of practice experience, gives us the base for diagnosis. Our range of different theories enriches this common core and provides us with further insights to help us understand and connect to clients in a manner that permits us to respond in an ethical, efficient, knowledge-based, helpful way.

# Chapter 13

# Diagnosis and the Computer

As I begin this chapter, I am struck quite forcibly with a non sequitur. I am working in a library that only allows pencils, not pens, to be used for handwritten work. This is a very old library in England where famous and ancient manuscripts are kept. However, in addition to pencils, personal computers are now permitted. Yet here I sit writing on foolscap, in pencil, about the potential of computers for the future of social work practice, surrounded by scholars of every discipline pouring over ancient manuscripts and making notes on Macintosh PowerBooks, which I have failed to bring with me.

The original title for this chapter was going to be "Diagnosis by Computer." As it began to take shape, I realized that what I wanted to present was not a technical chapter on the use of the computer as an aid to diagnosis. Others have begun this work and carried it forward. Rather, I wanted to craft a more speculative presentation on how the concepts of diagnosis and the power of this technology could come together.

Although we in social work long resisted the powerful resources for practice offered by the diverse range of readily available technologies, this period appears to be over. As a profession, we have advanced from a stage where many of us needed urging to consider the potency of these resources for our clients to a stage of attempting to keep up with the almost daily new uses in practice that are reported in our information exchange media. Certainly, although the development of this wide range of new practice resources is uneven, it seems we can stop urging their use in a hortative manner. Rather, we can now turn to the exciting task of evaluating and experimenting with their different uses.

Perhaps one reason we have not been more assiduous in specifying our diagnostic judgments in our records has been that we have lacked the resources to facilitate the process of setting out in an organized way the profile of judgments we make during the life of each case. The ability of the computer to organize, analyze, categorize, and correlate large quantities of diverse data in a rapid fashion may be the resource that will permit us to strengthen our diagnostic acumen. Increasing access to the omnipresent computer presents a powerful resource that would, and I argue should, enhance our diagnostic skills.

I have only made some tentative steps in considering the implications of the computer for practice. Others have gone further, and I hope that the utility of computers for the diagnostic component of practice will expand the ideas presented in the next few pages. What follows now is a summary of my thinking about some of the directions in which we might go with this resource.

Several of the computer's attributes appear highly relevant to the process and recording of diagnosis. First, of course, is the potential of the computer to store, sort, and retrieve material in a myriad of combinations and in an unbelievably short time. This attribute permits us to rapidly find and compare similar material from large collections of case files.

Many potential conceptual and practice payoffs for us stem from this capability. For example, we could look at similar diagnoses or similar attributes of diagnoses and compare them to interventions and outcomes. We could examine in a much richer way than we have done hitherto the question of how diagnoses formed from similar or diverse theoretical orientations impact on interventions and outcomes.

Computers would let us search for patterns of diagnosis in populations of practitioners, that is, what types of variables are always addressed, sometimes addressed, or never addressed. They also have the potential to reveal patterns of diagnoses between settings or between different groups of practitioners.

Exciting as this may sound, it is also daunting, for there is no magic about gathering and storing all this information in order to retrieve it. To gather and store it in a way in which it can be useful is hard work, time consuming, and expensive.

It should be possible to develop a range of options for each of the basic judgments that we make. These options could be further structured into a series of questions or prompts by a computer that would flag areas we had not covered in a diagnostic process and prompt us on possible alternative decisions we would need to consider.

If we moved in this direction, we would make considerable progress in the development of a much more standardized vocabulary than we have now. The diversity of terminology stemming from various theoretical orientations creates a particularly difficult challenge in efforts at extracting data from case records or in discussion with practitioners. To ensure, though, that the development of such a vocabulary does not cause rigidity, it is possible to construct computer programs that permit a broad and diverse vocabulary that would be sensitive to alternative usages.

Another aspect of a computer-assisted diagnosis would be ongoing testing of our levels of certitude about various aspects of a presenting situation and how such levels shift through the life of a case. In a similar way, prompts could be given in regard to the objectives of the case along with indications as to when they have changed.

Diagnostic aids that would facilitate a broad and diverse method of dealing with large quantities of data to help us organize our perceptions of cases from the perspective of treatment could also serve as powerful teaching aids. For example, by abstracting from a broad range of cases that contain very thorough and rich material, we could build simulated cases from which judgments could be made about what is known, what is critical, and what is relevant. These diagnoses could be formulated by students and evaluated. This is similar to what we do with case examples in the classroom. But by developing case simulations on the computer, students would be able to test their skills, enhance their skills, experiment with alternatives, ask for further information, and get instant feedback on their decisions and reactions to cases.

Clearly, I do not view the computer as a potential prescriber of intervention. Diagnosis provides a basis for certain actions; it does not tell us what actions to take. It is here that the richness of our theoretical base becomes operative. Although it is probably true that some presenting client situations do require some specific response, these are few in number. It appears that practitioners using different theories, viewing the world from different value sets, using different techniques, and practicing in different settings can be differentially yet powerfully effective.

The constant is that our client Mrs. Murphy is Mrs. Murphy no matter how we see her theoretically or diagnostically. Here the principle of equifinality from systems theory is critical. The actions we take with the client depend on many factors, including, of course, what the client wants and needs. But whatever we decide to do in particular situations needs to be related to our judgments and conclusions about the client, on which we have based our mutual setting of objectives with the client.

However, I can envisage computer programs that would alert us to possible risks in proceeding in particular directions. Also, considerable practice wisdom indicates that particular theoretical models are not appropriate for particular client value profiles or problem types. These data could be included in our programming as red flags or alerts to the therapist.

In no way am I suggesting that the computer will ever perform diagnosis or develop treatment plans in a prescriptive manner, as we dreamed in earlier decades, that treatment typologies for particular classifications of clients would do. What we can expect, however, is that a computer can prompt us to think about factors and clusters of factors that we may not have considered, alert us to changes in our view of a situation during a case, or prompt us to think about patterns of intervention or resources that might be helpful, or that are best avoided.

A further contribution could be envisaged in the development of diagnostic models. One way to proceed might be to develop a set of ten case summaries and put them on Web pages, then invite colleagues from anywhere in the world to formulate and submit diagnoses for these examples. One could then use qualitative and quantitative techniques to analyze the diagnoses submitted, out of which models could be developed. This would be a first step in developing formats that could serve as models of diagnosis. Only if we begin to develop such models for social work diagnoses and move to some increased commonality of viewpoint, style, and content will we be able to begin to identify what aspects of our intervention are effective and what are not.

All of this perhaps sounds very vague and without substance, but perhaps that is where we are in our practice. Certainly there are settings where diagnosis is part of the expected format of any case. In such settings, frequently the diagnosis is driven by the rigors of the

DSM paradigm. Of course, in many fields of practice our colleagues need an advanced level of DSM knowledge, but this conceptual body can only serve as one component of a social work diagnosis.

The power of the social work diagnosis is that it must seek to take into account the entire spectrum of a client's biopsychosocial purview. It is because of this complexity and breadth that I urge social workers to make use of the powerful, inexpensive, and widely available computer to help us move forward in this area of practice.

What the computer can and will do for us is to permit us to gather, manipulate, examine, and formulate profiles from large quantities of data across many variables in very short time spans. However, this is much easier to write about than to do. If we choose to march down this path in a much more aggressive and comprehensive way than before, we must be aware that the programming challenges are immense, though they are well within the potential of available resources. Other disciplines have learned to deal with vast amounts of data and huge numbers of subjects in manners that permit the building and manipulating of models and the identification of patterns. These in turn help advance the specific body of knowledge involved. We also can do this if the will is there.

As a first step I am suggesting (and hope to implement in the very near future) that we develop a Web site on which persons will be invited to submit examples of social work diagnoses, suitably disguised of course for the protection of the clients involved. This will permit us to begin content analysis for essential and common variables and their quantification. (The question of sharing diagnostic and case summary material is particularly difficult in social work. The challenge of ensuring that a case summary and diagnosis are sufficiently disguised to ensure confidentiality yet not to change the essence of the situation is complex and perhaps more risky than we have considered.)

The development of a body of data to permit us to begin to generalize on what social work diagnoses comprise is, as has been stated earlier, only a first step. In no way does it touch on the question of the relationship between diagnosis, intervention, and outcome. Such questions, of course, must be addressed, but the basis on which actions or interventions are taken needs to come first. Knowledge stemming from outcome evaluation supports our convictions that clients are helped and are pleased and satisfied with what happens to them in social work treatment. Our challenge now is to compare these favorable outcomes with what happened to clients in treatment and begin to ask much more specific questions about the helping process. Such as, do different styles or formats of intervention result in different outcomes?

Of course, I believe they do and build the concept of ethical and accountable practice on this. However, is what we do with clients based on our judgments about them or do each of us develop our own idiosyncratic profile of intervention that is applied to virtually every case? That is, do we all develop an "intervention for all occasions"? If this is what happens, then the concept of individual diagnosis is not nearly as critical as has been suggested in this book, except to ensure that we do not miss situations where serious harm can occur, or where we lack the competence to function adequately.

My argument, of course, is that the decisions we make about or with a client should be essentially related to what we do with, for, and to them, which in turn will affect the outcome. To adequately, effectively, and efficiently begin to address these questions as a profession will depend on a skillful use of the power of the computer. No longer is this a question of curiosity, or only within the purview of the academic researcher or those colleagues who have particular interest in computers. Rather, the issues and the potentials for enhancing our impact on clients are so great and the technical resources so available and powerful that all social workers need a sophisticated level of computer literacy. My fear is that some in the profession may see some type of dichotomy between the power of the helping relationship and the power of the microchip. Once we can begin to join these two powerful forces together, the potential positive impact on those we serve is almost impossible to comprehend.

I began the first draft of this chapter in longhand but thankfully have completed it on a computer. I hope this is symbolic of where we are in our profession. Over the decades, we have written much about the nature and necessity of diagnosis, but the time has now come to make use of available resources to move into a new era of careful study and analysis of this essential component of social work treatment.

# Chapter 14

# The Risks of Diagnosing

Diagnosis is risky in a variety of ways. It is risky for the client, and this is the most critical factor in this discussion. For if we are wrong in our diagnosis, even when the process involves a high degree of client participation, harm could occur. We know all too well that we can cause harm ranging from a mild inconvenience to a client to death, either of the client or someone else. Thankfully, life-and-death diagnostic errors are not a daily event for most of us. However, they do occur. The decision to leave a child in a particular situation can lead to his or her death through avoidable neglect, as can a misjudgment of a client's level of depression, which can lead to suicide. We can also misjudge a situation that can result in murder. In addition, and more frequently, misdiagnosis can deprive clients of available resources, techniques of intervention, the application of helpful theoretical models, and can cause misuse of treatment modalities, all of which can cause hurt at all degrees of severity. At a less serious level, a misdiagnosis can waste our time and our clients' time.

Rarely in our practice does a misdiagnosis have dramatic and cataclysmic results. For the most part, except in specialized situations, our clients are well-functioning persons whose difficulties lie in some aspect of their interactions with others, or in problems caused by some aspect of society's failures. However, it is because we see so many persons whose troubles are external to them rather than internal that we may miss those situations where the person is in critical shape.

Of course, misdiagnosing can result in harm to ourselves, as when a seriously upset person turns his or her anger on us. Unfortunately, a very real component of contemporary practice is the possibility of clients doing physical harm to therapists. This topic of worker safety, rarely if ever mentioned in schools of social work until about a decade ago, is now almost universally addressed in professional schools. Our state of knowledge is not at a level where we can always accurately judge the risk of harm from particular clients. However, it is such that we need to be aware of the possibility and at a minimum include it in the cluster of judgments we make throughout the diagnostic process.

Diagnosing is also risky because of its potential impact on the reputation of practitioners. To the extent that we seek to make precise diagnoses in relation to the client unit for which we are taking responsibility, it is possible for others to evaluate our work. Highly diffuse diagnoses may protect us from criticism (Kadushin 1963a), but such diffuseness also minimizes preciseness and efficiency in our practice.

When diagnosis is given a low priority, there is a tendency to vagueness in practice. This is not too serious when all is going well. It is of particular concern, however, when things have not gone well and there are few clear data as to what diagnostic judgments were the basis for intervention. It is this style of practice that rightfully causes criticism that we are only warmhearted do-gooders.

Thus, both incorrect diagnosing and failure to diagnose are risky. However, an incorrect diagnosis presents the opportunity to take corrective actions and to build knowledge both for ourselves and the profession. We, like those in all professions, learn as much from our mistakes and misdiagnoses as from correct diagnoses. I suggest that we do the most harm, and are thus most culpable, in those situations where there is no observable diagnosis. Although for a long time we have been able to get away with very sloppy, or indeed nonexistent diagnosis, society is no longer prepared to accept this.

Increasingly, our professional licensing and certifying bodies, insurance companies, our colleagues in other professions, the public, and, most important, our clients are expecting social workers to clearly state the conclusions that were the basis for their actions. Thus, the diagnostic process is going to become more risky, with higher expectations of precision from our clients, our colleagues, our agencies, other professions, our funders, and society.

But our practice has always been risky, as we have dared to intervene in the lives of persons and in the systems in which they live. In an earlier day it was much easier to hide our mistakes, and to fail to recognize bad and harm-creating practice. Any dramatic increase in accountability hinges on our ability to demonstrate that we know what we are doing, that is, on our ability to diagnose accurately and to intervene in a safe, effective way.

There appear to be at least three principal kinds of risk for practitioners in the diagnostic process. The first stems from a simple but critical lack of knowledge. I refer to mistakes we make just because we do not have sufficient knowledge about some aspect of a client's life or situation, or knowledge about existing resources, theories, techniques, or strategies. The humbling point is that we shall never know all we would want to know about social work practice. The challenge is to ensure that we have a level of knowledge that is in keeping with our profession's and society's reasonable expectations.

The second kind of risk in diagnosing is to either oversimplify or overcomplicate situations. The old scholastic Latin admonition *in media stat virtus* serves us well here. One of the reasons the concept of diagnosis came into disrepute in the late 1960s was the tendency to view client situations as extremely complex. We thought we needed to gather vast amounts of information about each client before we could commit ourselves to a helping process. This, of course, resulted in a Hegelian pendulum swing from thesis to antithesis. We moved to a restricted perception of treatment in which clients were seen in a much less complex perspective, and their problems for the most part were viewed as difficulties in daily living rather than flaws in their psychodynamic maturation. We now appear to be moving back to a realization that many clients really do only need some problem-solving or task-centered help, or some brief crisis work, but we are also seeing an increasing number of highly damaged and frail persons with limited internal or external resources. Such clients require the highest level of diagnostic knowledge and skill to understand them, connect to them, and engage them in a therapeutic process or help them connect to the resources they need.

We ought not view our practice purview as one situation or the other but as a spectrum on which we need to be ready to place ourselves at any point, at any time, and in any setting. If all a client needs is the opportunity to think and feel his or her way through a challenge in daily living, then that is what we should provide. If, on the other hand, a client requires two or three years of intense relationship therapy, involving not only our skills but those of other disciplines, that is what we need to provide. One treatment is not better than the other. The measure of a treatment's value rests on the accuracy of our diagnosis and our skill in responding in an appropriate, economic, client-responsive, therapeutic way.

The third risk in diagnosing is similar to the previous discussion in that the issues too often take the form of a dichotomy. This issue is probably a subset of the previous topic. I refer to the risk of over-pathologizing or depathologizing situations. We need to avoid being pushed into either extreme.

Without attempting to review the whole interrelated history of the mental health movement and the role of social work, psychiatry, and psychology, the terms *diagnosis* and *psychopathology* unfortunately became highly interconnected. As has been mentioned, in current practice this shows itself in the very common viewpoint that diagnosis means the use of the DSM. My thesis is that for social work the specificity of the DSM is important, but probably only for a very small percentage of our cases, apart from specialized mental health settings.

For the most part, our clients do not fit into any DSM classification unless the DSM in its future revisions finds a way to include every human being in some axis or category. (This excludes the DSM authors, of course.) But just because the majority of our clients are well-functioning persons does not mean we do not diagnose. To decide in a fifteen-minute phone call that a client only needs and wants information about the hours of service of a particular setting requires as much diagnostic knowledge and skill as it does to judge in a very few minutes that in fact this is a highly suicidal adolescent who needs the full gamut of our community's response mechanisms to save his life. We have to find our way between an antipathology perspective of clients and an all-encompassing perception that if we do not uncover some aspect of pathology, we have failed to make a "real" diagnosis. Unfortunately, when diagnosis became identified with a search for pathology in a psychiatrically oriented perspective, it lost its true meaning, which led to its rejection.

One further risk in diagnosis is the temptation to let our egos interface with the diagnostic process. This can occur in two or three different ways. First, we may let our own stubbornness get in the way and lock ourselves into a particular diagnostic formulation that we like and are unwilling to modify in view of further assessments, information, or reformulation. Thus we fall into the trap of making the data fit the diagnosis rather than letting the diagnosis emerge from the ongoing process in which we keep alternative explanations on our conceptual tables.

This same risk is present in regard to our colleagues. A more subtle form of professional inflexibility can occur when a colleague has a different diagnostic perspective than we do. It is difficult to be wrong, and even more difficult to admit this to a colleague. In social work, we have not developed in a structured way the practice of the second opinion. Often, in dialogue with a colleague who has a different perspective, a new understanding of a client emerges quite different from our own perspective or our colleague's.

This tendency to stick to our own judgments about a client in the light of a differing opinion becomes even more tempting when the alternate opinion comes from a colleague in another profession. Often, diagnostic differences are the battlefield on which complex sociological, political, power, and turf struggles are waged. It is often the insights of another profession that help us get a clear picture in a case. Those of us who have been fortunate enough to practice in multidisciplinary teams with a high degree of trust and collegiality know how enriching this can be, both to our own learning in general and to our understanding of particular cases. However, we have to be aware of the risks that at times our wish to demonstrate our own diagnostic acuity may overshadow the responsibility to be precise and certain. In such instance, our clients can suffer. It is better to accept that we are always learning, often at the price of some non-life-threatening blows to our egos.

Diagnosis is risky. So are many aspects of our professional practice. But so too is driving a car or flying in an airplane. All professional practice is risky. This is why professions have an ongoing process of raising standards, enhancing competence, and insisting on licensing, registration, and accreditation. Unfortunately, in our profession, since we deal with so many relatively intact persons in many instances, the harm we can cause in not diagnosing accurately can go unnoticed.

It is easy to avoid diagnosing and hide behind the much less precise term *assessment*. But if we are indeed committed to ethical practice of the highest competence that seeks first to do no harm and second to provide the optimum combination of skill, knowledge, and resources to clients, then we must accept and live with the very great risks that stem from a commitment to both the record and the process of diagnosis in our social work practice.

# Chapter 15

# Diagnosis and Research:
# A Contemporary Challenge

Thus far in this volume, my arguments and exhortations have been based on history, tradition, conviction, rationalizing, enthusiasm, and concern. These may be sufficient to discuss a topic and to argue a position, but they are not sufficient to insist on changed professional behavior. To do this I must be able to present evidence that what is being espoused here results in more effective intervention with clients. This I cannot do because such data do not exist.

At best, I can set out a challenge and an argument for targeted research. The challenge that now faces us relates to the essential issue of the relationship between the judgments we make about clients and how they affect the professional actions we take, and how in turn these actions affect the outcome of a case.

For example, we may be astute, precise, and diligent in our ability and commitment to formulate precise diagnoses of clients but find that these have little influence on what we choose or contract to do with them. That is, it may be that some of us develop tried and true patterns of intervention that make use of a very narrow cluster of theory, technique, methods, and resources with all clients. Hence, there may be little relationship between diagnosis and intervention. In such instances, there may be little difference in the pattern of intervention between a social worker who is as precise as possible in diagnosis and one who eschews the concept of diagnosis and practices only from a spontaneous emotion-based response to clients. In fact, from a research perspective, the possibility that the nondiagnosing colleague is more effective than one who diagnoses needs to be accepted.

My point is that to date, apart from our commitment to accountability in practice, from a research perspective we cannot make a strong case that diagnostic acumen and commitment are highly correlated with a good outcome. Certainly we know of more than a few examples of tragic outcomes in cases in which either no clear diagnosis or a misdiagnosis was made. Such cases, indeed, are sufficient to make a case for the correlation of diagnosis and intervention. However, life-and-death situations do not constitute the bulk of our practice. We must strive to assess if this correlation exists on a broader base.

Certainly, I believe that it does. As discussed in Chapter 2, for several decades it was the profession's clearly manifested position in our teaching, writing, and practice that diagnosis, treatment, and outcome were inextricably interwoven. In the present, all literature includes a position that some assessment process needs to be a part of every responsible professional intervention. However, from an empirical perspective we have not yet made a clear case for a correlation, and we must do so.

Much of the literature is written from a practice wisdom perspective. That is, it represents the reports of skilled colleagues on approaches to practice they have found useful in particular situations. In the myriad of diagnosis-based literature, there is yet a dearth of material that demonstrates that a minimal or nonexistent diagnosis results in a less effective outcome.

These questions are not raised in a spirit of cynicism or negativism. They are raised to urge us to pay more attention to the need to bring more precision to our practice. This in turn should enhance the ability to demonstrate our effectiveness. An important part of the thesis of this book is that we have let ourselves get so caught up in the sociology and politics of the terminology of diagnosis and the need for places to assign blame and criticism that we have not addressed the real issue of the need for a much greater degree of measurable precision in our work and in our outcomes.

But we ought not fall into the trap of name-calling and blaming those who may differ on the importance of diagnosis. Rather, we should start from a position of optimism, enthusiasm, and hopefully humility about the immensity of the task ahead of us.

Our profession has such a vast and highly diverse scope of interest, concern, and commitment that it is impossible for any one person to encompass the total spectrum of our practice. As our field of interests and concerns expands, so does the diversity of persons, situations, and resources and so does the body of our accumulated wisdom. We are living in a period of exciting, yet overwhelming, knowledge explosion. Certainly, when I first began to teach in the 1960s, it was possible to know the major literature and significant texts across a broad sweep of the profession. But a visit to the book display of any contemporary social work conference and a perusal of recent social work abstracts and research reminds us of the speed and volume of this knowledge base expansion.

These are exciting times. We have long since gotten over our defensiveness about our effectiveness. We know from both research and practice wisdom that we have a strongly positive impact. But we know that we do not help everyone. There are still many clients with whom we do not connect or whom we do not understand. Momentous societal problems remain to be faced. But this is true of all professions. Our strength now comes from a sense of the power of our knowledge and from the realization that we will advance knowledge in a slow, incremental process. This progress will not consist of major breakthroughs but small steps forward. We are doing much research of quality. Our literature reflects this. We once decried our lack of research; now we cannot keep up with even a small portion of it.

Another exciting factor is the great expansion of our ability to gather data on much larger bases and with much greater speed than used to be possible. Corresponding advances in analytic and statistical techniques permit us to manipulate both quantitative and qualitative data in a manner that lets us abstract small nuggets of fact from amounts of data. In particular, the differential influence of factors in complex situations can be more easily managed as we no longer attempt to see everything as linear, A causing B.

I urge that more of our contemporary and future research efforts be directed to the challenge of establishing to what extent diagnosis, treatment, and outcome are interconnected. This will not be done by major research efforts but though the accumulation of data from many small, structured projects carried out by small groups of colleagues in many diverse settings to begin to tease out the correlation of these factors.

If we begin to emphasize this research, I suggest that we not move too soon to regulate or attempt to standardize the form and content of diagnosis but welcome and attempt to learn from diversity. Each of us will have our own view of what a diagnosis should contain. I suggest that it is most important in this first wave of inquiry to put heavy stress on the recording of diagnosis, since in practice the process already exists. To date, our greatest problem in this area has been to find examples of what constitutes a social work diagnosis.

As discussed earlier, we do know what a diagnosis is not. But with the reality of a vast and diverse theoretical base of practice, with an inherently, broad range of differing vocabularies proper to each theory, it is inevitable that the perception of what words and ideas constitute a social work diagnosis will vary. Even in this diversity, it is important that we not be overly prescriptive as to format, as long as we agree that the aim of the record is to set out the judgments made by the social worker that serve as the basis for action. Once we have such records, we can begin to study them from the perspective of similarities and differences.

One of our challenges stems from a tradition that did not insist on precision and that too narrowly understood diagnosis. This is more complex in the current situation, where practice is driven by a broad spectrum of different theories. Hence we lack an internal agreed-upon, sanctioned lingua franca. Research is difficult in situations where we are attempting to examine and compare diagnoses from different perspectives.

From the viewpoint of vocabulary and different theoretical bases, there are several problems in doing research on diagnosis. In some situations, different theories use a similar vocabulary in discussing aspects of intervention but mean different things, for example the word *diagnosis* itself. In other situations, people use different vocabulary but mean similar things. For example, for some assessment is coterminous with diagnosis, although for others it describes a separate process. The third problem occurs when a particular theory introduces new vocabulary that describes phenomena known to other theories, such as, for example, the existential practitioners' preference for the word *encounter* instead of *relationship*. A fourth problem exists when both theories use the same vocabulary and mean the same things, but this is not recognized. There is a perception that terms must have different meanings if they come from different theoretical bases. Thus we need to tread cautiously, but not pessimistically, for such vocabulary and terminological challenges face all researchers.

Clearly some disciplines have greater consensus about terminology than social work has, but we are making progress. Several resources have emerged in recent decades that help move us to a common vocabulary. For example, the ongoing publication of the *Encyclopedia of Social Work* (1995) by the NASW and the emergence of similar volumes in other countries serve to enhance terminological consensus. In a similar way, the American-based *Social Work Dictionary,* edited by Dr. Robert Barker (1991), and its broad acceptance in the profession plays a major role as it establishes definitions of much of our terminology. Dr. Carlton Munson's (2000) recent volume on the DSM provides an excellent desk reference for describing and reporting mental health issues.

Although not written exclusively for social workers, a very helpful volume by Edward Zuckerman (1993) aims at producing a common language to describe a broad range of therapeutic situations. Further, the much-used DSM structures and the emerging PIE language specifically for social workers also play a similar role.

There are many other issues besides terminology and theoretical differences, but these are all manageable within the potential of today's resources. The critical point is that we should study many thousands of diagnostic records and learn what is essential to enhance treatment. Thus we have much to do, but the exciting point is that we have much to work from and many tools to use.

In summary, I believe the time is over for disputes about the validity of the term *diagnosis* or about how it is perceived. It is time to study how significant it is in the day-to-day work of frontline practitioners. Most important, we must begin to measure its implications for the quality of service we provide to clients.

# Chapter 16

# Enhancing Diagnostic Skills

If the reader who has come this far is in general agreement with the book's overall hypotheses, there should be support for the inclusion of a section on how to perform diagnosis more effectively.

The following ideas have not been tested but are suggestions for strategies that have been effective in enhancing other components of practice. They are thus seen as good places to start. The verb *start* is used advisedly to reflect the fact that we have written very little about how to diagnose more efficiently and effectively. We appear to presume that if a colleague understands the concept of diagnosis, he or she will know how to implement it in practice. Indeed, as a profession we have also written little on how to assess more effectively. I mention this lest some suggest that I have been blinded by my interest in diagnosis, that I have failed to take into account the work that has been done to enhance assessment skills.

My first suggestion is that we diagnose. That is, we should work to ensure that for each and every case there is a diagnosis.

I am assuming that one accepts the idea of a distinction between diagnosis and assessment. In many situations, the record includes a heading *assessment,* which frequently contains diagnosis-like judgments. By distinguishing between the two, I suggest we do a much better job of pushing ourselves to identify our judgments about which aspects of a client's life we have assessed as the basis for the selected pattern of intervention.

One other thing I have noticed is that assessments frequently read as succinct summaries of the clients' significant data and history. Often these are rich, and one gets a good sense of who the client is, but with little or no way of knowing which material was used as the basis of intervention.

In my days as a doctoral student at Columbia, our casework professor, Lucile Austin, used to drill us in writing diagnoses by having us write only a single paragraph, in which we were to include as succinctly as possible our opinions of the critical aspects of various cases with which we were presented. The paragraph was to begin, "This is a case of . . ." I have used this exercise with many classes of students and have found it to be an effective way to help students clarify the critical judgments they have made as to both strengths and concerns and how they fit together in a way that leads to some possible, feasible, and appropriate strategies of intervention in relation to what the client appears to want.

A related method of improving diagnostic skill is to work with peers in a "diagnosis improvement" project format, just as we do for various other kinds of professional enrichment. In such groups, we can take turns presenting a diagnosis of one of our cases and then answering questions about it posed by our colleagues. Two things can emerge from this type of activity. One, we can begin to see areas in the client's life where we have made judgments that have affected our actions but were not mentioned in our formal statements about them. We can also begin to see areas that we have overlooked or failed to assess, which may in turn affect the diagnosis. This is important, for as discussed in Chapter 8, we often make many decisions almost as reflexes or preconsciously and fail to appreciate how they direct or influence our subsequent actions.

Another important spin-off from such peer interaction is that we can both learn and teach each other ways of expressing our diagnostic judgments succinctly. Too often, especially for those who began to practice two or three decades ago, diagnostic statements include large amounts of historical and current information. We need considerable drill in succinctness, as our writing has not exemplified it much. Indeed, learning how to express a diagnosis is probably the most important outcome of peer groups and is one of the important ways that such peer groups are different from a case conference.

A further exercise that is useful in sharpening diagnostic skill is to work with colleagues in a format of collegial teaching. A very useful strategy is for a small group to take a case record and to have each person do a succinct diagnosis of it. These diagnoses are then compared on areas of agreement and disagreement. A common omission in such an exercise is a failure to report the conclusions. A useful way to begin is to use the list of critical judgments described in Chapter 8 to identify which judgments were reported, which appear to have been made and not reported, and which have not been made at all.

A commitment to the concept of diagnosis in social work practice is, of course, only a first step in ensuring that our clients receive the optimum care or intervention. Beyond the concept and the commitment, a multilayered strategy is required.

I think we would all improve our diagnostic skills if we ensured that several times throughout the life of a case we disciplined ourselves to write a diagnostic paragraph about it. In view of the complexity of today's practice, I am not certain we can always do this in a single paragraph, as Dr. Austin wished. I do think, though, that this type of exercise will bring us precision and accuracy.

I also suggest that students need opportunities to practice the diagnostic process. Certainly, in most social work programs considerable time is spent on case discussions, which indeed help students see relevant aspects of presenting situations along with areas they may have missed or misassessed. They also hear other perspectives and interpretations. What appears to be lacking in many instances is sufficient practice in learning to write succinct diagnoses from which precise plans of intervention are formulated.

Many practice settings are probably models of diagnostic practice in all its aspects. These we need to locate and make known. What concerns me is that few of our most frequently used methods textbooks give examples of diagnoses or assessments, if that is their concept of choice. We find frequent examples of summaries and descriptions of many components of cases but very few summarized statements that could stand as a diagnosis.

In this chapter, I have stressed the need to enhance our diagnostic acumen, but this cannot and must not become an end in itself. Just as there are serious risks in getting caught up in the "labeling game," we can fall into the "diagnostic game" in which we diagnose to show how wise we are, how our wisdom surpasses that of others, and to parade our journalistic prowess before others, especially members of another profession.

We must continually keep in mind that the only reason we diagnose is to better serve clients. The overarching challenge is to put a vast amount of energy into efforts to demonstrate the correlation between diagnostic acuity and outcome. For all our diagnostic efforts are in vain if we cannot show that more accurate diagnosis means a better outcome.

There is no easy road to make ourselves more consistent and effective diagnosticians. It is a part of the processes of which contemporary social work practice is composed. It is an expectation of our clients. It is an essential part of the responsibility and challenge we assume as social workers as we dare to intervene in the lives of individuals, dyads, groups, families, systems, and organizations.

# Chapter 17

# Final Comments

Although the idea for this work had been long generating, and the preliminary work was carried out in three countries, I did not start the actual writing until some four years ago. I do not recall the exact date on which I drafted the first outline, which has gone through many revisions, but I do know that it was shortly after returning from New York City where I had attended the 100th anniversary of Columbia University's School of Social Work, which marked as well the 100th anniversary of the beginning of professional social work in the United States.

The many historical papers presented there included frequent references to Mary Richmond, with emphasis on the importance of her 1917 work *Social Diagnosis*. I knew that it would be impossible for me to write about diagnosis in social work without reference to this seminal volume. However, I presumed that I would only need to make passing reference to it out of academic politeness and historical correctness. It had been many years since I had looked at this book (I noted on the inner front cover that I had purchased it for $1.00 many years ago). In reviewing it, I was most impressed with the extent to which Richmond had matured over the years and how up-to-date she had become. As I struggled with the ideas expressed in these chapters, it became very evident to me that this early colleague had a clear perception of the nature of diagnosis in social work, of its unique qualities in our profession, of its need to have a distinct purview separate from its use in other professions, and of our ethical responsibility to make it part of our practice. Three quotes from this work stood out for me:

> In social diagnosis there is the attempt to arrive at as exact a definition as possible of the social situation and personality of the client. (p. 51)

There would be few more dangerous things than a social diagnosis that was not subject to review in the light of further facts. (p. 361)

Last of all, full diagnosis—any correct diagnosis in fact—is not always possible, even when there is ample time. We are dealing with human factors and we too are human. . . . Be it repeated no diagnosis is final. Since later developments in a case may clarify the social practitioner's insight into its causal factors, there is a sense in which investigation continues as long as treatment. (p. 373)

The original title for this book was to be *Social Work Diagnosis.* However, as the various chapters began to take shape, I began to understand that rather than a work on how to diagnose, my primary interest was to examine how and why in our first hundred years we had let the concept drift from its original status as a basic root of our practice to be rejected by many. Thus, the book that did emerge is rather a dissertation which argues that the time has come to readdress this issue with the hope of getting us back on the trail of enhancing our diagnostic skills for the good of our clients.

As mentioned earlier, I began with the arrogant presumption that I was going to be the only person carrying this flag of truth. I was to "fight the impossible fight," as did the Man of La Mancha. However, as I began to examine this issue further and to discourse with my colleagues in several countries, my sense of being the lonely champion was quickly eradicated. For, as several times alluded to earlier, a most important finding for me was that the concept and practice of diagnosis was not moribund, but alive and well in many parts of the profession, especially among experienced frontline clinicians. Thus my quest has become a less ambitious one, which is to urge that those who have eliminated the term and concept of diagnosis from their personal professional lexicons at least revisit the issue.

As I write these final pages, I ask myself, What then are my realistic hopes and aspirations for this book? First I put aside any fantasy that the content of these pages is so compelling that there will be a rush to rescue social work diagnosis from its misdirected wanderings and unfair exile. Rather, I hope that at least a few colleagues will put the matter on the table for further examination and discussion.

If we could at least see the term *psychosocial diagnosis* as neutral, then we could put more effort into the most critical aspect of this discussion: does it really matter? Rather than debate word usage, let us put tangible efforts into testing, through the myriad strategies now available to us, whether a commitment to, and acuity in, the process and recording of diagnosis lead to more effective interventions and reduced misinterventions. This is really the only thing that matters in this discussion.

Thus, I urge that consideration be given to the following six possible actions:

1. Authors of social work methods and practice texts should present a more balanced view of the concept of diagnosis and its place in our present practice. To continue to use a misdefinition of diagnosis and thereby reject it is hardly the mark of quality scholarship.

2. The editors of the most valuable and influential *Encyclopedia of Social Work* should reintroduce in the next edition an entry on diagnosis similar to the one as they presently have on assessment. The weight of evidence shows that this is still a powerful concept in the profession and cannot be ignored. Hence, so prestigious a set of volumes as this encyclopedia owes it to the profession to at least present diagnosis as a concept that is alive and well in significant components of the profession, even though somewhat battered.

3. Additional research should be carried out that addresses the history, sociology, and politics of social work diagnosis in the past and present in a much more thorough and scholarly way than has been done up to now.

4. We should begin to develop networks of scholars, practitioners, and clinical scientists who can debate, study, and work to implement a more positive and aggressive approach to diagnosis in day-to-day practice as well as in the development and testing of theory and its impact on clients.

5. Encouragement should be given to research projects that focus on testing, in both small and large projects, the interface of diagnosis, intervention, and outcome.

6. Those of us entrusted with the awesome responsibility of shaping our future colleagues should ensure that we present at least a balanced view of the assessment/diagnosis dialogue in our teaching. Further, whether or not we still decide to favor the term *as-*

*sessment* over *diagnosis,* we should emphasize the ethical need for precision in building our interventions with clients on the basis of the judgments we make about them.

Throughout this book, the word *client* has been used as if it referred only to a single person. This was done for ease in writing, for of course client can mean individuals, dyads, families, groups, or communities. Obviously it is much easier to talk about a client as a singular entity, and indeed much of this book sounds as if it is only single clients whom we diagnose.

Complex as is the process of diagnosis of a single person, it is much more so for multiple clients. But we cannot despair nor be daunted by the immensity of our task. Colleagues in other disciplines such as astronomy or physics have faced equally complex conceptual challenges and have mastered huge masses of intervening variables similar to the one we first identified as a discrete term, "person-in-situation." Other disciplines have been struggling with theoretical (read diagnostic) challenges for centuries.

We need not hope to do everything in one century. Remember that the search for a solution to the challenge of measuring longitude, so critical to navigation, took several centuries, yet is a process we take for granted in our very commonplace airplane and sea voyages today. The important thing is that the challenge was recognized, faced, and ultimately conquered.

Thus far in social work we seem to have addressed the daunting diagnostic challenge by changing its name in the hope that it will go away. It will not, no matter what we call it. We must accept enthusiastically, yet humbly, the diagnostic challenge and stumble along with it as did our colleagues in other disciplines until in some future day we will hone our currently crude skills in a manner that will ensure a more efficient and effective service to clients.

Helen Harris Perlman has said that no matter what our theory or theories of practice, and no matter what we call the process, we all diagnose. Florence Hollis took it as a given that diagnosis was the essence of responsible practice. With assertions such as this by some of the luminaries of our profession, then it appears we have only two alternatives. The first is to deny or ignore these admonitions by prolonging a misinterpretation of the meaning of diagnosis and continuing the word game of substitution.

The second is to accept this importance of the term as a starting point of our deliberations and reinstate diagnosis to at least a point of neutrality so that we can examine its import, content, place, risk, and challenges in our daily practices. In so doing, we can continue to implement our mission of bringing to bear the total impact of our accumulated body of knowledge, skill, resources, techniques, experience, and wisdom to guarantee that the services we offer are safe, individualized, ethical, effective, and economic and offered in a manner that ensures that no harm is done.

# Appendix

# Some Examples
# of Social Work Diagnoses

In the following pages, five examples of a possible format for social work diagnosis are presented. These are not real cases or modified cases but have been created as examples of the kinds of situations
a social worker might meet in a general service agency. Thus, any re-
semblance to real cases or people is entirely coincidental.

I decided to make up these cases rather than use disguised real
cases because of the real challenge of ensuring that colleagues, students, or clients would not wonder if I was using material from a case
they knew. In crafting these examples, I tried to include material that
reflected the areas of judgment that were discussed in Chapter 8.

## Case 1*

Based on the material presented in a first interview, in my opinion
this twenty-eight-year-old single Caucasian heterosexual male of
Irish/French descent appears to be in good mental and physical
health. He is of average or slightly above average intelligence. Although he has shown some low-level outbursts of anger with friends,
he does not appear to be a person who will engage in assaultive behavior, nor are there any indications of suicidal thoughts. He communicates well in a quiet, introspective, believable manner. Although
not practicing his religion, he has a strong or even oversevere con-
science. He is strongly identified with his French-Canadian origins,
which appears to be a source of considerable stress in his job. His personal and social network, although not extensive, is strong, varied,

---

*Cases 1, 2, and 3 are from F. Turner (Ed.) 1999. *Social Work Practice: A Canadian
Perspective.* Toronto: Allyn & Bacon, pp. 129-130. Cases 4 and 5 are original to this book.

and supportive. He is experiencing a moderate level of stress with respect to the stability of his employment, which is further exacerbated by a rather large number of debts that he appears to be managing.

The major area of concern for which he is seeking help relates to a strong sense of uncertainty as to his life direction. He would benefit from a brief series three to four of one-to-one interviews aimed at helping him look at his strengths and alternatives from a Gestalt perspective. I think he will benefit considerably from this and will not require any further assistance.

*Source:* F. Turner (Ed.) (1999). *Social Work Practice: A Canadian Perspective.* Toronto: Allyn and Bacon, pp. 129-130.

## Case 2

Mrs. G. is a seventy-five-year-old woman of Chinese/East Indian origins, recently arrived from Ghana and living with her eldest daughter and family. The following stems from a series of four interviews, in two of which Mrs. G.'s daughter was present.

It appears that this woman is in good mental health but that her several physical problems related to arthritis and accompanied by a complex regime of medication have resulted in a slight restriction of spontaneity—the seriousness of which is greatly exaggerated by the daughter.

Her strong but small network of friends give her considerable support, as do her close associations with both the spiritual and social functions of her church. The very limited financial situation of the family appears to be under control and not affecting the mother-daughter relationship. Mrs. G. contributes much to the family as a skilled housekeeper and handiwoman.

The mild level of observed depression, confirmed by her physician, does not represent any threat to her. It is viewed by her physician as situationally caused, and I agree.

Mrs. G. would like to feel more respected and appreciated and less infantilized by her daughter. The daughter appears to be a highly intact person, quite comfortable in looking at her interaction and considering modifications in it. Both are prepared to look at themselves and came to the agency with the strong urging of their pastor. The daughter is somewhat uncertain about the role of the agency and the nature of psychosocial treatment and will need some further learning in order to make full use of the relationship and our services.

This is a situation that could become more serious if the mother-daughter relationship deteriorates. However, with a present-centered supportive ongoing relationship, some role changes in both the mother and daughter appear possible. It may be that, in the future, an educationally focused self-help group of women newly arrived from other countries could further help the daughter better understand her own and her mother's psychosocial situation in a new country. I would view the prognosis of this situation as moderately positive.

*Source:* F. Turner (Ed.) (1999). *Social Work Practice: A Canadian Perspective.* Toronto: Allyn and Bacon, pp. 129-130.

### Case 3

Mr. G. is a twenty-eight-year-old Caucasian Canadian born of Polish/Scottish parents. He has been medically treated for a diagnosed moderately severe schizophrenic condition since age seventeen, for which a carefully monitored program of medication permits him to function moderately well in the community. He appears to be of above-average intelligence and highly gifted and interested in music. He is no threat to himself or others, although at times his severely bizarre behavior, consisting mostly of verbal hallucinations, is of considerable stress to his family, who have still not fully accepted or understood his condition. Nevertheless, his family is available to him, and they are strongly supportive of him, but not in a knowledgeable way.

He has few friends or acquaintances but is able to effectively use the network of services available in the community. He handles his money, provided by his family, reasonably well, although he is frequently criticized by his mother for what she views as irresponsibility in traveling to concerts of interest to him or purchasing expensive audio equipment.

In my opinion, from a case management perspective, this young man will be able to function for many years living on his own. The approach should stress the provision of concrete services and problem-solving approaches as needed. He is not a person with whom close therapeutic relationship should be attempted, nor should he be invited to join a group. Rather, he will do well by knowing and being known by a service network composed of many helpful and available but not intrusive persons.

*Source:* F. Turner (Ed.) (1999). *Social Work Practice: A Canadian Perspective.* Toronto: Allyn and Bacon, pp. 129-130.

## Case 4

Mr. F. is a highly intelligent forty-five-year-old recent immigrant from Eastern Europe, well educated and multilingual, with no serious financial problems and a comfortable, steady income as an interpreter, a position in which he takes considerable pride. He states he is and appears to be in good physical and mental health and is not on any medication. He was originally referred here by his physician, as he wanted an opportunity to sort out with "a professional therapist" an important life decision in regard to a contemplated marriage. He communicates well in a clear, convincing manner in a style in which he speaks to himself more than directly to me.

He is a quiet, private, soft-spoken, reserved person, highly introspective, with a small but close-knit circle of highly supportive friends, both male and female, with common interests in art and culture in general.

He has strong guilty feelings about his marriage plans, the source of which are unclear to me at this point, but which appear to be related to his being an only son and having left his widowed mother in the old country.

He related quickly to me and is comfortable and interested in looking at his history and its relationship to his current dilemma. He now appears to be at a point where he can free himself from his past and move forward in his current life plans. He has benefited and should continue to benefit considerably from this relationship, in which I have given him considerable support in his self-reflection, with some challenging of his own self-interpretations. The relationship need not move beyond its present level of reflective consideration and should not be long term. I have now seen him three times and plan to have two more interviews to, as he says, "finish cleaning up the past."

It is clear that he has made great strides in freeing himself from his earlier history and has gained considerable insight about himself, although I do not fully understand some of this material and its meaning for him. The prognosis for this situation is highly positive.

## Case 5

Miss P. is a well-groomed, slightly built, twenty-eight-year-old single mother of Oriental origin with a two-year-old mixed-race child. A friend in her apartment, a former client, referred her to the agency. She described serious difficulties with her landlord, who was threatening eviction. She appears to be of average or perhaps slightly less intelligence and is in good mental and physical health apart from taking medication for high blood pressure. She is attentive to her medication and makes regular visits to a neighborhood clinic. She has completed high school, is working part-time in a department store, and is taking a food preparation course downtown. She appears to be an attentive, responsible, caring mother. She is a highly impulsive person with strong mood swings and mentioned in a matter-of-fact manner that in the past she has had occasional suicidal thoughts when things were going badly for her. I believe she has a very traumatic history but she is not interested in talking about it.

She related very guardedly and slowly. She is a problem solver and is here to find a solution to her problem with the landlord. She is a future-oriented person determined to move ahead in her life. She has sufficient resources to live on, aided by both financial and emotional support from her father, who lives in a distant city and maintains phone contact with her. She has an active social life but no regular boyfriend at this time. She was raised a Catholic, and although she has minimal contact with her church, this is a part of her identity. From my first contact with her I have an opinion that she is not fully believable, with a tendency to embellish the facts of a situation. Although as our relationship developed she did seem to want to talk about herself, she made it clear that she only wanted to work on her problem with the landlord and, apart from my discomfort as to her veracity, I do believe she is functioning well at this time.

Based on a letter from her landlord that she showed me and her own description of the situation, it was clear that she does have a problem in regard to her tenancy but had not thought of legal assistance. She eagerly accepted a referral to a lawyer available to the agency as well as my offer to accompany her for her first visit, as she showed some anxiety about meeting a lawyer. The visit went well and the lawyer was able to straighten the matter out, to her great satisfaction.

She has since called the agency from time to time to "chat." I encourage this, as I am still very uncertain as to her overall stability and how she would function in a more precarious situation. At this point, I am confident that she takes good care of her child but not so sure as to her own functioning.

# Bibliography

Abramovitz, R. and Williams, J. B. W. (1992). Workshop 2: The pros and cons of the Diagnostic and Statistical Manual for social work practice and research. *Research on Social Work Practice,* 2(3), 338-349.

Ackerman, N. W. (1961). A dynamic frame for the clinical approach to family conflict. In L. Beatman and S. Sherman (Eds.), *Exploring the base for family therapy* (pp. 52-67). New York: Family Service Association of America.

Altmeyer, J. (1956). Public school services for the child with emotional problems. *Social Work,* 1(1), 96.

American Psychiatric Association (1994). *Diagnostic and statistical manual of mental disorders* (Fourth edition). Washington, DC: Author.

Anello, E. (1989). DSM-III is a useful tool: Response to Kutchins and Kirk. *Social Work,* 34(2), 186-188.

Aptekar, H. H. (1939). Diagnosis: A changing concept. In F. Lowry (Ed.), *Readings in social case work, 1920-1938* (pp. 249-257). New York: Columbia University Press.

Aptekar, H. H. (1955). *The dynamics of casework and counseling.* Boston: Houghton Mifflin.

Axelrod, P., Cameron, M., and Soloman, J. C. (1944). An experiment in group therapy with shy adolescent girls. *American Journal of Orthopsychiatry,* 14, October 616-627.

Badri, M. B. (1967). A new technique for the systematic desensitization of pervasive anxiety and phobic reactions. *The Journal of Psychology,* 65, (second-half) 201-208.

Bahn, A. (1965). Need of a classification scheme for the psychosocial disorders. *Public Health Reports,* 80, January 79-82.

Bahn, A. K., Chandler, C. A., and Eisenberg, H. (1961). Diagnostic and demographic characteristics of patients seen in out-patient psychiatric clinics for an entire state: Implications for a psychiatrist and the mental health program planner. *American Journal of Psychiatry,* 117, March 769-778.

Banes, L. (1961). Direct casework treatment of a latency-age child. *Social Casework,* 42(4), 124-137.

Barker, R. L. (1991). *The social work dictionary.* Silver Spring, MD: National Association of Social Workers.

Barnes, M. (1965). Casework with children. *Smith College Studies in Social Work,* 35(3).

Barnwell, J. (1960). Group treatment of older adolescent boys in a family agency. *Social Casework*, 41, 247-253.

Beatman, F. L. (1957). Family interaction: Its significance for diagnosis and treatment. *Social Casework*, 38(3), 111-118.

Beck, B. (1958). The adolescent's challenge to casework. *Social Work*, 3(2), 89-95.

Becker, D. A. (1966). Casework for the aged poor: A renewed drive for public-voluntary teamwork. *Social Casework*, 47(5), 293-301.

Begab, M. J. (1964). Counselling parents of retarded children. *Canada's Mental Health*, 12(3), 2.

Berg, R. (1964). Utilizing the strengths of unwed mothers in the AFDC program. *Child Welfare*, 43(7), 333-339.

Berkowitz, S. (1955). Some specific techniques of psychosocial diagnosis and treatment in family casework. *Social Casework*, 36(9), 399-406.

Berleman, W. C. (1968). Mary Richmond's social diagnosis in retrospect. *Social Casework*, 49, 395-402.

Bernard, J. (1959). *Social problems at midcentury: Role status, and stress in a context of abundance*. New York: Dryden Press.

Bernstein, R. (1960). Are we still stereotyping the unwed mother? *Social Work*, 5(3), 22-38.

Birchard, C. (Ed.) (1964). Prevention of mental illness and social maladjustment. *Canada's Mental Health*, Special Supplement, 44, ii-23.

Bloch, J. B. (1968). The white worker and the Negro client in psychotherapy. *Social Work*, 13(2), 36-42.

Block, H. I. (1958). Casework services in a geriatric clinic. *Social Casework*, 39(4), 228-235.

Bloom, M. L. (1973). Usefulness of the home visit for diagnosis and treatment. *Social Casework*, 54(2), 67-75.

Boehm, W. (1962). Diagnostic categories in social casework. *Social Work Practice: 1962 National Conference on Social Welfare* (pp. 3-26). New York: Family Service Association of America.

Bonan, F. A. (1963). Psychoanalytic implications in treating unmarried mothers with narcissistic character structures. *Social Casework*, 44(1), 323-329.

Briar, S. (1976). Toward autonomous social diagnosis. *Bulletin of the Menninger Clinic*, 40(5), 593-601.

Brown, L. B. (1950). Race as a factor in establishing a casework relationship. *Social Casework*, 31(3), 91-97.

Bruck, M. (1966). An evaluation of the use of group treatment for "hard-to-reach" latency-age children in a community guidance clinic. *Child Welfare*, 45(7) 395-403.

Bruck, M. (1968). Behavior modification theory and practice: A critical review. *Social Work*, 13(2), 43-55.

Butterfield, W. H. (1986). Computers in Social Work and Social Welfare: Issues and Perspectives. *A Journal of Sociology and Social Welfare* 9(1), 5-26.

Caplan, P. J. (1992). Gender issues in the diagnosis of mental disorder. *Women and Therapy: A Feminist Quarterly,* 12(4), 71-82.

Caplan, P. J. (1995). *They say you're crazy: How the world's most powerful psychiatrists decide who's normal.* Reading, MA: Addison-Wesley.

Carleton, T. O. (1989). Classification and diagnosis in social work in health care. *Health and Social Work,* 14(2), 83-85.

Carson, R. (1967). A and B therapist "types": A possible critical variable in psychotherapy. *The Journal of Nervous and Mental Disease,* 144(1), 47-53.

Caughlan, J. (1960). Psychic hazards of unwed paternity. *Social Work,* 5(3), 29-35.

Chaiklin, H. (1974). Social work, sociology, and social diagnosis. *Journal of Sociology and Social Welfare,* 2(1), 102-107.

Chance, E. (1963). Implications of interdisciplinary differences in case description. *American Journal of Orthopsychiatry,* 33 (July), 673-677.

Cheek, F. E. (1965). Family interaction patterns and convalescent adjustment of the schizophrenic. *Archives of General Psychiatry,* 13(2), (August) 138-147.

Christmas, J. J. (1967). Sociopsychiatric treatment of disadvantaged psychotic adults. *American Journal of Orthopsychiatry,* 37(1), 93-100.

Chwast, J. (1966). The resocialization of the discharged depressed patient. *Canadian Psychiatric Association Journal,* 11, Supplement, 131-140.

Clifton, E., and Hollis, F. (Eds.) (1948). *Child therapy: A Casework Symposium.* New York: Family Service Association of America.

Cohen, R. G. (1957). Casework with older persons. *Social Work,* 2(1), 30-35.

Colcord, J. C. (1919). *Broken homes: A study of family desertion and its social treatment.* New York: Russell Sage Foundation.

Collins, A. and Mackay, J. (1959). Casework treatment of delinquents who use the primary defense of denial. *Social Work,* 4(1), 34-43.

Colt, A. (1967). Casework treatment of a borderline client. *Social Casework,* 48(8), 482-488.

Compton, B. R. and Galaway, B. (1989). *Social work processes.* Homewood, IL: Dorsey Press.

Confer, C. E. and Lessor, L. R. (1967). Preventative mental health groups for the aged. *Lutheran Social Welfare Quarterly,* 1.

Courtenay, W. (1991). Are borderline clients underidentified in social agencies? *Clinical Social Work Journal,* 19(3), 309-325.

Cowden, R. C. and Ford, L. I. (1962). Systematic desensitization with phobic schizophrenics. *American Journal of Psychiatry,* 119, (September) 241-245.

Crammer, L. (1961). Treatment and fashion in treatment. *American Journal of Psychiatry,* 118, (November) 447-448.

Curfman, H. G. and Arnold, C. B. (1967). A homebound therapy program for severely retarded children. *Children,* 14(2), 63-68.

Cutler, C. E. (1991). Deconstructing the DSM-III. *Social Work,* 36(2), 154-157.

Cutter, A. V. and Hallowitz, D. (1962). Different approaches to treatment of the child and parents. *American Journal of Orthopsychiatry,* 32(1), 152-158.

Darke, R. E. and Mueser, K. T. (Eds.) (1996). *Dual diagnosis of major mental illness and substance abuse.* San Francisco: Jossey-Bass.

Davitto, B. and Scullion, T. (1967). An experiment in community treatment of delinquents. *Social Casework,* 48(1), 10-16.

Dawes, R. M. (1994). *House of cards: Psychology and psychotherapy built on myth.* New York: Free Press.

Dawley, A. (1937). Diagnosis—the dynamic of effective treatment. *Journal of Social Work Process,* 1(1), 19-31.

Denton, W. (1990). A family systems analysis of DSM-III-R. *Journal of Marital and Family Therapy,* 16(2), 113-125.

Devis, D. A. (1967). Four useful concepts for family diagnosis and treatment. *Social Work,* 12(3), 18-27.

Distler, L. S., May, P. R., and Hussain, S. T. (1964). Anxiety and ego strength as predictors of response to treatment in schizophrenic patients. *Journal of Consulting Psychology,* 28(2), 170-177.

Dorfman, R. A. (Ed.) 1988. *Paradigms of Clinical Social Work.* New York: Brunner/Mazel.

Drake, R. E. and Mueser, K. T. (1996). *Dual diagnosis of major mental illness and substance abuse* (Volume II). San Fransisco: Jossey-Bass.

Driekurs, R. (1963). Psychodynamic diagnosis in psychiatry. *American Journal of Psychiatry,* 119, (May) 1045-1048.

Ehrenkranz, S. M. (1967). A study of joint interviewing in the treatment of marital problems: Part I. *Social Casework,* 48(8), 498-501.

Eidelberg, L. (1956). Neurotic choice of mate. In V. Eisenstein (Ed.), *Neurotic interaction in marriage* (pp. 57-64). New York: Basic Books.

Eisenberg, M. S. (1956). Psychodynamic aspects of casework with the unmarried mother. In *Casework papers* (pp. 71-90). New York: Family Service Association of America.

*Encyclopedia of Social Work,* Nineteenth edition, (1995) R. Edwards, (Ed.). Washington, DC: NASW Press.

Enelow, A. J. (1960). The silent patient. *Psychiatry,* 23, 153-158.

Eysenck, N. J. and Rachman, S. (1965). *The causes and cures of neuroses.* London: Routledge and Keegan Paul.

Ferdinand, B. (1963). Psychoanalytic implications in treating unmarried mothers with narcissistic character structures. *Social Casework,* 44(6), 323-329.

Fertel, P. and Reiss, R. E. (1997). Counselling prenatal diagnosis patients: The role of social work. *Social Work in Health Care,* 24(3-4), 47-63.

Finck, G. H., Reiner, B. S., and Smith, B. O. (1965). Group counseling with unmarried mothers. *Journal of Marriage and the Family,* 27(2), 224-229.

Finestone, S. (1960). Issues involved in developing diagnostic classifications for casework. In *Casework papers* (pp. 139-154). New York: Family Service Association of America.

Finlayson, A. D. (1937). The diagnostic process in continuing treatment. *Social Casework,* 18(7), 228-233.

Finn, S. E. (1982). Base rates, utilities, and DSM-III: Shortcomings of fixed-rule systems of psychodiagnosis. *Journal of Abnormal Psychology,* 91(4), 294-302.

Fischer, J. (1970). Portents from the past: What ever happened to social diagnosis? *International Social Work,* 13(2), 18-28.

Flesch, R. (1949). The problem of diagnosis in marital discord. *Social Casework,* 30, 355-362.

Ford, C. S. (1965). Ego adaptive mechanisms of older persons. *Social Casework,* 46(1), 16-21.

Freeman, H., Hildebrand, C., and Ayre, D. (1965). A classification system that prescribes treatment. *Social Casework,* 46(7), 423-429.

Frey, L. A. and Kolodny, R. L. (1966). Group treatment for the alienated child in the school. *International Journal of Group Psychotherapy,* 16(3), 321-337.

Friedman, H. L. (1966). The mother-daughter relationship: Its potential in treatment of young unwed mothers. *Social Casework,* 47(8), 502-506.

Fuller, T. K. (1970). Computer utility in social work. *Social Casework,* 51(10), 606-611.

Funtowicz, M. N. and Widiger, T. A. (1995). Sex bias in the diagnosis of personality disorders: A different approach. *Journal of Psychology and Behavioural Assessment,* 17(2), 145-165.

Furnari, J., et al. (1967). Casework treatment techniques and clinical diagnosis: A study of their relationship in the casework interview. Unpublished master's thesis, Graduate School of Social Work, Adelphi University.

Gabriel, B. (1944). Group treatment for adolescent girls. *The American Journal of Orthopsychiatry,* 14, (October) 593-602.

Galdston Grunebaum, M. (1961). A study of learning problems of children: Casework implications. *Social Casework,* 42(9), 461-468.

Galdston Grunebaum, M., et al. (1962). Fathers of sons with primary neurotic learning inhibitions. *American Journal of Orthopsychiatry,* 32(3), 462-472.

Gambril, E. D. (1983). *Casework: A competency-based approach.* Englewood Cliffs, NJ: Prentice Hall.

Ganter, G. and Polansky, N. A. (1964). Predicting a child's accessibility to individual treatment from diagnostic groups. *Social Work,* 9(3), 56-63.

Ganter, G., Yeakel, M., and Polansky, N. (1965). Intermediary group treatment of inaccessible children. *American Journal of Orthopsychiatry,* 35(4), 739-746.

Garland, J. A., Kolodny, R. L., and Waldfogel, S. (1962). Social group work as adjunctive treatment for the emotionally disturbed adolescent: The experience of a specialized group work department. *American Journal of Orthopsychiatry,* 32(4), 691-706.

Garvin, C. and Glasser, P. (1970). The basis of social treatment. In *Social Work Practice,* 1970 National Conference on Social Welfare, NY: Columbia University Press, 149-177.

Gehrke, S. and Moxom, J. (1962). Diagnostic classifications and treatment techniques in marriage counseling. *Family Process,* 1(2), 253-264.

Gelder, M. G. and Marks, I. M. (1966). Severe agoraphobia: A controlled prospective trial of behaviour therapy. *British Journal of Psychiatry,* 112, (March) 309-319.

Gelfand, B. (1972). Emerging trends in social treatment. *Social Casework,* 53(3), 156-162.

Gellman, I. P. (1964). *The sober alcoholic: An organizational analysis of Alcoholics Anonymous.* New Haven: College and University Press.

Gitelson, M. (1948). Character synthesis: The psychotherapeutic problem of adolescence. *American Journal of Orthopsychiatry,* 18, (July) 422-431.

Glenn, M. L. (1984). *On diagnosis: A systemic approach.* New York: Brunner.

Gochros, J. S. (1966). Recognition and use of anger in Negro clients. *Social Work,* 11(1), 28-34.

Goldsmith, A. (1959). Challenges of delinquency to casework treatment. *Social Work,* 4(2), 14-19.

Goldsmith, J. (1950). Treatment of the adolescent girl with superego defect. *Social Casework,* 31(4), 139-145.

Golner, J. H. (1964). Learning problems and identity problems of latency-age boys. *Social Casework,* 45(9), 534-539.

Gomberg, M. R. and Levinson, F. T. (Eds.) (1951). *Diagnosis and process in family counselling.* New York: Family Service Association of America.

Goodman, E. M. (1968). Habilitation of the unwed teenage mother: An interdisciplinary and community responsibility. *Child Welfare,* 47(5), 274-280.

Goodman, L. (1964). Continuing treatment of parents with congenitally defective infants. *Social Work,* 9(1), 92-97.

*Guidelines for selection of treatment methods.* (1968). Family and Children's Services of Greater St. Louis.

Hallowitz, D. (1966). Individual treatment of the child in the context of family therapy. *Social Casework,* 47(2), 82-86.

Hallowitz, D. and Cutler, A. V. (1958). A collaborative diagnostic and treatment process with parents. *Social Work,* 3(3), 90-97.

Hamilton, G. (1937). Basic concepts in social case work. In F. Lowry (Ed.), *Readings in social case work, 1920-1938* (pp. 155-171). New York: Columbia University Press.

Hamilton, G. (1951). *Theory and practice of social case work.* New York: Columbia University Press.

Hamilton, G. (1955). Casework diagnosis. *Journal of Jewish Communal Services,* 31(3), 389-395.

Hamilton, G. (1963). *Psychotherapy in child guidance.* New York: Columbia University Press.

Harper-Dorton, K. and Herbert, M. (1998). *Working with children and their families* (Second edition). Chicago: Lyceum Books.

Harris, J. K. (1967). *Automating welfare: Potential and problems.* Santa Monica, CA: System Development Corporation.

Healy, W. (1915). *The individual delinquent: A text-book of diagnosis and prognosis for all concerned in understanding offenders.* Boston, MA: Little, Brown.

Hellenbrand, S. C. (1961). Client value orientations: Implications for diagnosis and treatment. *Social Casework, 42*(3), 163-169.

Hepworth, D. H. (1964). The clinical implications of perceptual distortions in forced marriages. *Social Casework, 45*(10), 579-585.

Hepworth, D. H. (1986). *Direct social work practice: Theory and skills* (Second edition). Chicago: Dorsey Press.

Hepworth, D., Rooney, R. H., Larson, J. (1997). Direct social work practice, Fifth edition. New York: Brooks Cole Publishing.

Hersh, A. (1961). Casework with parents of retarded children. *Social Work, 6*(2), 61.

Hersko, M. (1962). Group psychotherapy with delinquent adolescent girls. *American Journal of Orthopsychiatry, 32*(1), 169-175.

Herzog, E. (1966). Some notes about unmarried fathers. *Child Welfare, 45*(4), 194-197.

Hill, C. G. (1965). Alcoholism-therapy. *Addictions, 12*(2), 10-16.

Hogarty, G. E. (1966). The components of casework judgment. *Social Casework, 47*(3), 165-171.

Hollis, F. (1949). Women in material conflict. New York: Family Service Association of America.

Hollis, F. (1951). The relationship between psychosocial diagnosis and treatment. *Social Casework, 32*(1), 67-74.

Hollis, F. (1954). Casework diagnosis—What and why? *Smith College Studies in Social Work, 24*(3), 1-8.

Hollis, F. (1958). Personality diagnosis in casework. In H. J. Parad (Ed.), *Ego psychology and dynamic casework* (pp. 83-96). New York: Family Service Association of America.

Hollis, F. (1965). *Casework: A psychosocial therapy.* New York: Random House.

Hollis, F. (1968a). A profile of early interviews in marital counseling. *Social Casework, 49*(1), 35-43.

Hollis, F. (1968b). Continuance and discontinuance in marital counseling and some observations on joint interviews. *Social Casework, 49*(3), 167-174.

Hollis, F. (1970). A psychosocial approach to casework. In R. W. Roberts and R. H. Nee (Eds.), *Theories of social casework* (pp. 33-76). Chicago: University of Chicago Press.

Hollis, F. and Family Service Association of America (1968). *A typology of casework treatment.* New York: Family Service Association of America.

Hollis, F. and Family Welfare Association of America (1939). *Social casework in practice—Six case studies.* New York: Family Welfare Association of America.

Hopkins, J. (1978). Models of assessment in social work. *British Journal of Social Work, 8*(4), 465-475.

Howells, J. G. (1986). *Family diagnosis.* New York: International Universities Press.

Jacob, C. (1967). The value of the family interview in the diagnosis and treatment of schizophrenia. *Psychiatry,* 30, 162-172.

Jacobson, E. (1938). *Progressive relaxation.* Chicago: University of Chicago Press.

Jellineck, E. M. (1960). *The disease concept of alcoholism.* New Haven, CT: Hillhouse Press.

Johnson, A. and Fishback, A. R. (1944). Analysis of a disturbed adolescent girl and the collaborative psychiatric treatment of the mother. *American Journal of Orthopsychiatry,* 14(April), 195-203.

Johnson, H. (1988). Where is the border? Current issues in the diagnosis and treatment of the borderline. *Clinical Social Work Journal,* 16(3), 243-260.

Johnson, L. (1998). *Social work practice,* Sixth edition. Toronto: Allyn & Bacon.

Johnson, R. F. and Lee, H. (1965). Rehabilitation of chronic schizophrenics. *Archives of General Psychiatry,* 12(3), 237-240.

Jones, W. C., Meyer, H. J., and Borgatta, E. F. (1967). Social and psychological factors in status decisions of unmarried mothers. In E. J. Thomas (Ed.), *Behavioral science for social workers* (pp. 170-177). New York: The Free Press.

Jordan, C. and Franklin, C. (1995). Clinical assessment for social workers: Quantitative and qualitative methods. Chicago: Lyceum Books

Josselyn, I. (1966). *The adolescent and his world.* New York: Family Service Association of America.

Kadushin, A. (1963a). Diagnosis and evaluation for (almost) all occasions. *Social Work,* 8(1), 12-19.

Kadushin, A. (1963b). Testing diagnostic competence: A problem for social work research. *Social Casework,* 44(7), 397-405.

Kaplan, A. (1956). Psychiatric syndromes and the practice of social work. *Social Casework,* 37(3), 107-112.

Karet, S. and Harrington, B. (1958). An objective method for prediction of casework movement. *Social Work,* 3(4), 45-52.

Karls, J. W. and Wandrei, K. E. (1995). Person in Environment. In R. Edwards (Ed.), *Encyclopedia of Social Work,* Nineteenth Edition. Washington, DC: NASW Press.

Kasius, C. (1950a). A comparison of diagnostic and functional casework concepts. Report of the Family Service Association of America *"Committee to Study Basic Concepts in Casework Practice."*

Kasius, C. (Ed.) (1950b). *Principles and techniques in social casework: Selected articles, 1940-1950.* New York: Family Service Association of America.

Kasius, C. (Ed.) (1953). *Principles and techniques in social casework.* New York: Family Service Association of America.

Kaslow, F. W. (1993). Relational diagnosis: An idea whose time has come? *Family Process,* 32(2), 255-259.

Kaufman, I. (1958). Therapeutic considerations of the borderline personality structure. In H. J. Parad (Ed.), *Ego psychology and dynamic casework,* (pp. 99-110). New York: Family Service Association of America.

Kaufman, I. (1962). Maximizing strengths of adults with severe ego defects. *Social Casework,* 43(9), 478-485.

Keeney, B. P. (1979). Ecosystemic epistemology: An alternative paradigm for diagnosis. *Family Process,* 18(2), 117-129.

Kelley, F. (1965). Research in schizophrenia: Implications for social workers. *Social Work,* 10(1), 32-44.

Kent, A. (1965). *Specialized information centers.* Washington, DC: Spartan Books.

Kirk, S. A. and Kutchins, H. (1988). Deliberate misdiagnosis in mental health practice. *Social Service Review,* 62(2), 225-236.

Kirk, S. A. and Kutchins, H. (1992). *The selling of DSM: The rhetoric of science in psychiatry.* New York: Aldine de Gruyter.

Kirk, S. A. and Kutchins, H. (1994). The myth of the reliability of DSM. *Journal of Mind and Behavior,* 15(1-2), 71-86.

Kirk, S. A., Siporin, M., and Kutchins, H. (1989). The prognosis for social work diagnosis. *Social Casework,* 70(5), 295-304.

Kirst-Ashman, K. and Hull, G. Jr. (1993). *Understanding generalist practice.* Chicago: Nelson-Hall.

Kitchener, H., Sweet, B., and Citrin, E. (1961). Problems in the treatment of impulse disorder in children in a residential setting. *Psychiatry,* 24(4), 347-356.

Kline, M., Sydnor-Greenberg, N., Davis, W. W., Pincus, H. A., and Frances, A. J. (1993). Using field trials to evaluate proposed changes in DSM diagnostic criteria. *Hospital and Community Psychiatry,* 44(7), 621-623.

Klugman, D. J., Litman, R. E., and Wold, C. I. (1965). Suicide: Answering the cry for help. *Social Work,* 10(4), 43-50.

Konopka, G. (1963). *Social groupwork.* Englewood Cliffs, NJ: Prentice-Hall.

Konopka, G. (1966). *The adolescent girl in conflict.* Englewood Cliffs, NJ: Prentice-Hall.

Kotis, J. P. (1968). Initial sessions of group counselling with alcoholics and their spouses. *Social Casework,* 49(4), 228.

Kraft, T. and Al-Issa, H. (1965). The application of learning theory to the treatment of traffic phobia. *British Journal of Psychiatry,* 111 (March), 277-279.

Kramer, M., Koon, G., and Eisenberg, L. (1967). *World Health Organization diagnostic exercise.* Boston: Massachusetts General Hospital.

Krill, D. F. (1967). Loosening the Oedipal bind through family therapy. *Social Casework,* 48(9), 563-569.

Krill, D. F. (1968). A framework for determining client modifiability. *Social Casework,* 49(10), 602-611.

Kunst, M. S. (1959). Learning disabilities: Their dynamics and treatment. *Social Casework,* 4(2), 95-101.

Kutchins, H. and Kirk, S. A. (1986). The reliability of DSM-III: A critical review. *Social Work Research and Abstracts*, 22(4), 3-12.

Kutchins, H. and Kirk, S. A. (1987). DSM-III and social work malpractice. *Social Work*, 32(3), 205-211.

Kutchins, H. and Kirk, S. A. (1988). The business of diagnosis: DSM-III and clinical social work. *Social Work*, 33(3), 215-220.

Kutchins, H. and Kirk, S. A. (1989a). DSM-III-R: The conflict over new psychiatric diagnoses. *Health and Social Work*, 14(2), 91-101.

Kutchins, H. and Kirk, S. A. (1989b). Human errors, attractive nuisances, and toxic wastes: A reply to Anello. *Social Work*, 34(2), 187-188.

Lampe, H. (1961). Diagnostic considerations in casework with aged clients. *Social Casework*, 42(5-6), 240-244.

Lang, P. J. and Lazovick, A. D. (1963). Experimental desensitization of a phobia. *Journal of Abnormal and Social Psychology*, 66(6), 519-525.

Lantz, J. E. (1987). *An introduction to clinical social work practice.* Springfield, IL: Charles C. Thomas.

Laughlin, H. P. (1967). *Neuroses.* Washington, DC: Butterworth.

Lazarus, A. A. (1961). Group therapy of phobic disorders by systematic desensitization. *Journal of Abnormal and Social Psychology*, 63(3), 504-510.

Lehrman, L. J. (1954). The logic of diagnosis. *Social Casework*, 35(5), 192-199.

Lehrman, L. J. (1960). *Psychosocial diagnostic categories.* Pittsburgh: University of Pittsburgh, School of Social Work.

Leichter, E. and Schulman, G. L. (1968). The prevention of family break-up. *Social Casework*, 49(3), 143-150.

Leichter, H. J. (1961). Kinship values and casework intervention. In *Casework papers* (p. 58). New York: Family Service Association of America.

Levitt, E. E. (1963). Psychotherapy with children: A further evaluation. *Behavior Research and Therapy*, 1(1), 41-51.

Levy, S. (1981). Labeling: The social worker's responsibility. *Social Casework*, 62, 332-342.

Leyendecker, G. (1957). Generic and specific factors in casework with the unmarried mother. In National Conference on Social Welfare (Ed.) *Casework papers* (pp. 113-129). New York: Family Service Association of America.

Little, R. (1949). Diagnostic recording. *Social Casework*, 30(1), 15-19.

Longabaugh, R., Stout, R., Kriebel, G. W., McCullough, L., and Bishop, D. (1986). DSM-III and clinically identified problems as a guide to treatment. *Archives of General Psychiatry*, 43(11), 1097-1103.

Lowry, F. (1938). Current concepts in social case-work practice. *The Social Service Review*, 12(4), 571-597.

Lowry, F. (Ed.) (1939). *Readings in social case work, 1920-1938.* New York: Columbia University Press.

Mackey, R. (1976). Generic aspects of clinical social work practice. *Social Casework*, 57(10), 619-624.

Mackey, R. A. (1964). Family casework diagnosis by Alice Voiland and Associates. *International Journal of Group Psychotherapy,* 14(1), 123-124.

MacMillan, D. (1960). Community mental health: The Mapperley hospital scheme. *Canada's Mental Health,* Special Supplement.

Maeder, L. M. A. (1941). Diagnostic criteria—The concept of normal and abnormal. In C. Kasius (Ed.), *Principles and techniques in social casework: Selected articles, 1940-1950* (pp. 285-300). New York: Family Service Association of America.

Mahrer, A. R. (Ed.) (1970). *New approaches to personality classification.* New York: Columbia University Press.

Mandlebaum, A. (1967). The group process in helping parents of retarded children. *Children,* 14(6), 227.

Martin, J. M. (1957). Social-cultural differences: Barriers in casework with delinquents. *Social Work,* 2(3), 22-25.

Mason, E. M. (1968). The contribution of the social history on the diagnosis of child disturbances. *The British Journal of Psychiatric Social Work,* 9(4), 180-187.

Mattaini, M. A. and Kirk, S. A. (1991). Assessing assessment in social work. *Social Work,* 36(3), 260-266.

Mattaini, M. A. and Kirk, S. A. (1993). Misdiagnosing assessment. *Social Work,* 38(2), 231-233.

Mauney, F., Fox, M. E., and Vines, M. A. (1966). Tenth-grade girls and early marriage: A school-agency project. *Social Casework,* 47(2), 98-103.

Mayer, J., Myerson, D. J., Needham, M. A., and Fox, M. (1967). Treatment of the female alcoholic: The former prisoner. *American Journal of Orthopsychiatry,* 37(5), 932-937.

McLachlan, G. and Shegof, R. A. (Eds.) (1968). *Computers in the service of medicine* (Volumes I and II). London: Oxford University Press.

McPhatter, A. R. (1991). Assessment revisited: A comprehensive approach to understanding family dynamics. *Families in Society,* 72(1), 11-22.

McWhinnie, A. M. (1967). *Adopted children—How they grow up.* Don Mills, ON: General Publishing.

Meenaghan, T. M. and Gibbons, W. E. (1998). Generalist practice and skills in larger systems.

Meier, E. G. (1959). Social and cultural factors in casework diagnosis. *Social Work,* 4(3), 15-26.

Meyer, C. (1993). *Assessment in social work practice.* New York: Columbia University Press.

Meyer, C. H. (1992). Social work assessment: Is there an empirical base? *Research on Social Work Practice,* 2(3), 297-305.

Meyer, R. E., Schiff, L. F., and Becker, A. (1967). The home treatment of psychotic patients. *American Journal of Psychiatry,* 123(1), 1430-1438.

Meyer, V. (1957). The treatment of two phobic patients on the basis of learning principles. *Journal of Abnormal and Social Psychology,* 55, 261-266.

Meyer, V. and Gelder, M. G. (1963). Behavior therapy and phobic disorders. *British Journal of Psychiatry*, 109(1), 19-28.

Miller, L. (1965). Short-term therapy with adolescents. In H. J. Parad (Ed.), *Crisis intervention*. (pp. 157-166). New York: Family Service Association of America.

Miller, P. and Ferone, L. (1966). Group psychotherapy with depressed women. *American Journal of Psychiatry*, 123(6), 701-703.

Milloy, M. (1964). Casework with the older person and his family. *Social Casework*, 45(8), 450-456.

Mitchell, C. B. (1960). The use of family sessions in diagnosis and treatment of disturbance in children. *Social Casework*, 41(6), 283-290.

Moorhead, M. (1937). What is involved in simplicity of treatment? In F. Lowry (Ed.), *Readings in social case work, 1920-1938* (pp. 258-267). New York: Columbia University Press.

Morrison, J. R. (1995). *DSM-IV made easy: The clinician's guide to diagnosis*. New York: Guilford Press.

Moynihan, F. M. (1968). Data processing in the administration of a family agency. Family Service Highlights, 29(3), 67-73.

Mulinski, P. (1989). Dual diagnosis in alcoholic clients: Clinical implication. *Social Case Work*, 70(6), 333-339.

Mullen, E. J. (1969). The relation between diagnosis and treatment in casework. *Social Casework*, 50(4), 218-226.

Munson, C. E. (2000). *The mental health diagnostic desk reference*. Binghamton, NY: The Haworth Press.

Nadal, R. (1961). Counseling program for parents of severely retarded pre-school children. *Social Casework*, 42(2), 78-83.

Nadeau, K. G. (Ed.) (1995). *A comprehensive guide to attention deficit disorder in adults: Research, diagnosis, and treatment*. New York: Brunner/Mazel.

Nathan, P. E. (1967). *Cues, decisions, diagnosis*. New York: Academic Press.

National Social Welfare Assembly (1962). *The impact of racial factors on casework services*. Report of the Intergroup Relations Clinic. New York: Author.

Nichols, W. C. and Rutledge, A. L. (1965). Psychotherapy with teenagers. *Journal of Marriage and the Family*, 27(2), 166-171.

Nurius, P. S. and Hudson, W. W. (1989). Computers and social diagnosis: The client's perspective. *Computers in Human Services*, 5(1-2), 21-35.

Ogren, E. H., Norris-Shortle, C. A., and Showalter, A. (1979). Typologies in social work practice. *Social Work in Health Care*, 4(3), 319-330.

O'Neil, M. J. (1990) *The general method of social work practice*, Second edition. Englewood Cliffs, NJ: Prentice-Hall.

Oppenheim, J. (1991). *"Shattered nerves": Doctors, patients, and depression in Victorian England*. New York: Oxford University Press.

O'Rourke, H. and Chavers, F. (1968). The use of groups with unmarried mothers to facilitate casework. *Child Welfare*, 47(1), 17-25.

Ostrower, R. (1962). Study diagnosis and treatment: A conceptual structure. *Social Work*, 7(4), 86-91.

Pannor, B., Evans, B., and Massarick, F. (1967). Standardized case recording in casework practice and research: The "SCRF" as a tool in the study of unwed parenthood. *Child Welfare*, 46 (December), 569-574.

Pannor, R. and Evans, B. (1967). The unmarried father: An integral part of casework services to the unmarried mother. *Child Welfare*, 46, 150-155.

Panter, E. J. (1966). Ego-building procedures that foster social functioning. *Social Casework*, 47(3), 139-145.

Parad, H. and Miller, R. (Eds.). (1963). *Ego-oriented casework: Problems and perspectives*. New York: Family Service Association of America.

Parad, H. J. (1965). A framework for studying families in crisis. In Parad (Ed.) *Crisis intervention* (pp. 53-75). New York: Family Service Association of America.

Parker, E. B., Olsen, T. F., and Throckmorton, M. C. (1960). Social casework with elementary school children who do not talk in school. *Social Work*, 5(2), 64-70.

Pasamaniek, B. (1963). On the neglect of diagnosis. *American Journal of Orthopsychiatry*, 33, (April) 397-398.

Pattison, E. M. (1967). Abstinence criteria in alcoholism treatment. *Addictions*, 14(3), 1-19.

Peck, H. and Bellsmith, V. (1965). *Treatment of the delinquent adolescent: Group therapy and individual therapy with parent and child*. New York: Family Service Association of America.

Perlman, H. H. (1956). The client's treatability. *Social Work*, 1(4), 32-40.

Perlman, H. H. (1957). *Social casework: A problem solving process*. New York: Family Service Association of America.

Perlman, H. H. (1962). The role concept and social casework: Some explorations: II. What is social diagnosis? *Social Service Review*, 36(1), 17-31.

Perlman, H. H. (1968). *Persona: Social role and personality*. Chicago: University of Chicago Press.

Perlman, H. H. (1970). The problem-solving model in social casework. In R. W. Roberts and R. H. Nee (Eds.), *Theories of social casework* (pp. 129-180). Chicago: University of Chicago Press.

Pharis, M. E. (1967). The use of adolescents' creative writing in diagnosis and treatment. *Social Casework*, 48(2), 67-74.

Philips, I. (Ed.) (1966). *Prevention and treatment of mental retardation*. New York: Basic Books.

Phillips, D. C. (1960). Of plums and thistles: The search for diagnosis. *Social Work*, 5(1), 84-90.

Pieper, M. (1989). The heuristic paradigm: A unifying and comprehensive approach to social work research. *Smith College Studies in Social Work*, 60(1), 8-34.

Pinderhughes, E. (1989). *Understanding race, ethnicity and power: The key to efficacy in clinical practice*. New York: Free Press.

Polansky, N. A. (1967). On duplicity in the interview. *American Journal of Orthopsychiatry,* 37(3), 568-579.

Pollak, O. (1952). Age-sex roles and psychotherapy of adolescents. In O. Pollak (Ed.) *Social science and psychotherapy for children* (pp. 133-147). New York: Russel Sage Foundation.

Pollak, O. and Brieland, D. (1961). The Midwest seminar on family diagnosis and treatment. *Social Casework,* 42(7), 319-324.

Pollak, O., Young, H. M., and Leach, H. (1960). Differential diagnosis and treatment of character disturbances. *Social Casework,* 41(10), 512-517.

Pope, H. (1967). Unwed mothers and their sex partners. *Journal of Marriage and the Family,* 29(3), 555-567.

Prugh, D. (1970). Psychosocial disorders in childhood and adolescence: Theoretical considerations and an attempt at classification. Appendix A in *Child Mental Health: Challenge for the 1970's.* Report of the Joint Committee on Mental Health of Children. New York: Harper and Row.

Pruyser, P. W. and Menninger, K. (1976). Language pitfalls in diagnostic thought and work. *Bulletin of the Menninger Clinic,* 40(4), 417-434.

Rabichow, H. (1963). Casework treatment of adolescents with learning inhibitions. *Social Work,* 8(4), 55-62.

Raffoul, P. R. and Holmes, K. A. (1986). DSM-III content in social work curricula: Results of a national survey. *Journal of Social Work Education,* 22(1), 24-31.

Rank, O. (1936). *Will therapy.* New York: Knopf.

Rapoport, L. (1970). Crisis intervention as a mode of treatment. In R. W. Roberts and R. H. Nee (Eds.), *Theories of social casework* (pp. 265-312). Chicago: University of Chicago Press.

Regan, P. F. (1965). Brief psychotherapy of depression. *American Journal of Psychiatry,* 122, July, 28-32.

Reid, J. D. (1983). *Diagnosis and intervention in behavior therapy and behavioral medicine.* New York: Springer.

Reiner, B. and Kaufman, I. (1959). *Character disorders in parents of delinquents.* New York: Family Service Association of America.

Ressler, T. J. (1994). Quality care for individuals with dual diagnosis. The legal and ethical imperative to provide qualified staff. *Mental Retardation,* 32(5), 356-361.

Reynolds, B. (1951). Is diagnosis an imposition. In *Social work and social living.* New York: Citadel Press.

Richmond, M. E. (1917). *Social diagnosis.* New York: Russell Sage Foundation.

Richmond, M. E. (1922). *What is social casework? An introductory description.* New York: Russell Sage Foundation.

Richmond, M. E., et al. (1930). *The long view: Papers and addresses by Mary E. Richmond.* J. C. Colcord (Ed.). New York: Russell Sage Foundation.

Ripple, L., Alexander, E., and Polemis, B. (1964). *Motivation, capacity and opportunity.* Chicago: University of Chicago Press.

Roberts, R. W. and Nee, R. H. (Eds.) (1970). *Theories of social casework.* Chicago: University of Chicago Press.

Robinson, V. (1930). *A changing psychology in social case work.* Chapel Hill, NC: University of North Carolina Press.

Rodwell, M. K. (1987). Naturalistic inquiry: An alternative model for social work assessment. *Social Service Review,* 61(2), 231-246.

Rogers, C. (1951). *Client-centered therapy.* Boston: Houghton Mifflin.

Rosenblatt, A. and Woldfogel, D. (1983). *Handbook of clinical social work.* Washington, DC: Jossey-Bass.

Rosenfeld, S. K. and Sprince, M. P. (1963). An attempt to formulate the meaning of the concept borderline. *Psychoanalytic Study of the Child,* 18, 603-635.

Rowan, M. and Pannon, R. (1959). Work with teen-age unwed parents and their families. *Child Welfare,* 38(10), 16-21.

Ruffin, W., Goggins, D., and Dowis, J. (1965). Milieu and the schizophrenic patient. *Archives of General Psychology,* 12(5), 516-519.

Saari, C. (1980). Contributions from linguistics to an understanding of affect in diagnosis and treatment. *Clinical Social Work Journal,* 8(4), 223-235.

Saari, C. (1986). *Clinical social work treatment.* New York: Gardner Press.

Saari, C. (1994). An exploration of meaning and causation in clinical social work. *Social Work Journal,* 22(3), 251-261.

Sackheim, G. (1974). *The practice of clinical casework.* New York: Behavioral Publications.

Sacks, S. P. (1949). Establishing the diagnosis in marital problems. *Social Casework,* 30(5), 181-187.

Sainsbury, E. E. (1970). *Social diagnosis in case work.* London: Routledge.

Satir, V. (1967). *Conjoint family therapy.* Palo Alto, CA: Science and Behavior Books.

Savage, N. J., Weltman, R., and Zarfas, D. E. (1967). Short-term care for the mentally retarded. *Mental Retardation,* 5(2), 9-14.

Scarbrough, H. E. (1968). The hypothesis of hidden health in the treatment of severe neurosis. *Social Casework,* 49(3), 294.

Scheidlinger, S. (1966). The concept of latency: Implications for group treatment. *Social Casework,* 47(6), 363-368.

Scheiner, S. (1964). On the therapy of schizophrenia. *The American Journal of Psychoanalysis,* 23-24, 167-183.

Scherz, F. (1971). Maturational crises and parent-child interaction. *Social Casework,* 52(6), 362-376.

Scherz, F. H. (1970). Theory and practice of family therapy. In R. W. Roberts and R. H. Nee (Eds.), *Theories of social casework* (pp. 219-264). Chicago: University of Chicago Press.

Scheunemann, Y. R. and French, B. (1974). Diagnosis as the foundation of professional service. *Social Casework,* 55(3), 135-141.

Schild, S. (1964). Counselling with parents of retarded children living at home. *Social Work*, 9(1), 86-91.

Schuckit, M. A. (1995). *Drug and treatment abuse: Clinical guide to diagnosis and treatment.* New York: Plenum Medical Book.

Seaberg, J. R. (1965). Case recording by code. *Social Work*, 10(4), 92-96.

Selby, L. G. (1958). Typologies for caseworkers: Some considerations and problems. *Social Service Review*, 32(4), 341-349.

Sheer, R. M. and Sharpe, W. M. (1965). Group work as a treatment. *Mental Retardation*, 3(3), 23-25.

Sherman, E. and Reid, W. (Eds.) (1994). *Qualitative research in social work.* New York: Columbia University Press.

Sherman, S. (1966). Family treatment: An approach to children's problems. *Social Casework*, 47(6), 368-372.

Shipman, G. (1959). Probation and the family. In S. Glueck (Ed.), *The problem of delinquency* (pp. 618-623). Boston: Houghton Mifflin.

Sholtis, H. S. (1964). The management of marital counseling cases. *Social Casework*, 45, 71-78.

Sibulkin, L. (1959). Special skills in working with older people. *Social Casework*, 40(4), 208-212.

Simcox, B. R. (1947). Diagnostic process in marital problems. *Social Casework*, 28(8), 307-313.

Simmons, L. C. (1963). Crow Jim: Implications for social work. *Social Work*, 8(3), 24-30.

Simon, B. K. (1970). Social casework theory: An overview. In R. W. Roberts and R. H. Nee (Eds.), *Theories of social casework* (pp. 353-398). Chicago: University of Chicago Press.

Simons, R. L. and Argner, S. M. (1985). *Practice principles: A problem-solving approach to social work.* New York: Macmillan.

Siporin, M. (1970) Social treatment: A new-old helping method. *Social Work*, 15(3), 13-25.

Skidmore, R. A. and Van Streeter Garrett, H. (1959). The joint interview in marriage counseling. *Journal of Marriage and the Family*, 17(4), 349-354.

Skodol, A. E. (1989). Problems in differential diagnosis: From DSM-III to DSM-III-R in clinical practice. Washington, DC: American Psychiatric Press.

Slavson, S. (1964). *A textbook in analytic group psychotherapy.* New York: International Universities Press.

Slavson, S. R. and MacLennan, B. (1956). *Unmarried mothers: The fields of group psychotherapy.* New York: John Wiley and Sons.

Smalley, R. E. (1956). The school social worker helps the troubled child. *Social Work*, 1(1), 103-108.

Smalley, R. E. (1967). *Theory for social work practice.* New York: Columbia University Press.

Smalley, R. E. (1970). The functional approach to casework. In R. W. Roberts and R. H. Nee (Eds.), *Theories of social casework* (pp. 77-128). Chicago: University of Chicago Press.

Smith, D. and Kraft, W. A. (1983). Do psychologists really want an alternative? *American Psychologist*, 38(7), 777-785.

Solomon, A. (1992). Clinical diagnosis among diverse populations: A multicultural perspective. *Families in Society: The Journal of Contemporary Human Services*, 73(6), 371-377.

Spearman, F. W. and Vesper, S. (1966). Treatment of marital conflict resulting from severe personality disturbance. *Social Casework*, 47(9), 583-589.

Sperry, B., Ulrich, D. N., and Stover, N. (1958). The relations of motility to boys' learning problems. *American Journal of Orthopsychiatry*, 28, July, 640-646.

Sperry, L. (1995). *Handbook of diagnosis and treatment of the DSM-IV personality*. New York: Brunner/Mazel.

Stites, M. A. (1958). Psychosocial diagnosis in vocational rehabilitation services. *Social Casework*, 39(1), 21-27.

Strean, H. S. (1967). Role theory, role models, and casework: Review of the literature and practice applications. *Social Work*, 12(2), 77-88.

Strean, H. S. (Ed.) (1971). *Social casework: Theories in action*. Metuchen, NJ: Scarecrow Press.

Strean, H. S. (1974). Choosing among practice modalities. *Clinical Social Work Journal*, 2(1), 3-14.

Stuart, R. (1964). Supportive casework with borderline patients. *Social Work*, 9(1), 38-44.

Stuart, R. B. (1967). Casework treatment of depression viewed as an interpersonal disturbance. *Social Work*, 12(3), 27-36.

Sytz, F. (1948). The development of method in social casework. In C. Kasius (Ed.), *Principles and techniques in social casework: Selected articles, 1940-1950* (pp. 314-323). New York: Family Service Association of America.

Taft, J. (1937). The relation of function to process in social casework. *Journal of Social Work Process*, 1(1), 1-18.

Taft, J. (Ed.) (1944). *A functional approach to family case work*. New York: Columbia University Press.

Taussig, H. P. (1939). Treatment as an aid to diagnosis. *Social Casework*, 19(9), 289-294.

Taylor-Brown, S. (1995). HIV/AIDS: Direct practice. In R. Edwards (Ed.) *Encyclopedia of Social Work* (Nineteenth Edition, Volume 2, pp. 1291-1305). Washington, DC: NASW Press.

Tharp, R. G. (1965). Marriage roles and family treatment. *American Journal of Orthopsychiatry*, 35(2), 531-538.

Thomas, D. V. (1951). The relationship between diagnostic service and short-contact cases. *Social Casework*, 32(2), 74-81.

Thomas, E. J. (1968). Selected sociobehavioral techniques and principles: An approach to interpersonal helping. *Social Work,* 13(1), 12-26.

Thomas, E. J. (1970). Behavioral modification and casework. In R. W. Roberts and R. H. Nee (Eds.), *Theories of social casework* (pp.181-218). Chicago: University of Chicago Press.

Thomas, J. R. (1994). Quality care for individuals with dual diagnosis: The legal and ethical imperative to provide qualified staff. *Mental Retardation,* 32(5), 356-365.

Towle, C. (1941). Underlying skills of case work today. *Social Service Review,* 15(3), 456-471.

Turner, F. (Ed.) (1996). *Social work treatment,* Fourth edition. New York: Free Press.

Turner, F. (Ed.) (1999). *Social work practice: A Canadian perspective.* Toronto: Allyn and Bacon.

Turner, F. J. (1968). *Differential diagnosis and treatment in social work.* New York: The Free Press.

Turner, F. J. (1969). The search for diagnostic categories in social work treatment. Paper presented at the Learned Societies of Canada, York University, Toronto, Ontario, Canada.

Turner, F. J. (1978). *Psychosocial therapy: A social work perspective.* New York: Free Press.

Turner, F. J. (1986). Psychosocial theory. In F. J. Turner (Ed.), *Social work treatment: Interlocking theoretical approaches* (Third edition, pp. 484-513). New York: Free Press.

Turner, F. J. (1994). Reconsidering diagnosis. *Families in Society,* 73(March), 168-171.

Turner, F. J. (1995). *Differential diagnosis and treatment in social work* (Fourth edition). New York: Free Press.

Turner, H. (1961). Use of the relationship in casework treatment of the aged. *Social Casework,* 42(5-6), 245-251.

Twente, E. E. (1965). Aging, strength and creativity. *Social Work,* 10, 105-110.

Tyler, E. A., Trumaa, A., and Henshaw, P. (1962). Family group intake by a child guidance team. *Archives of General Psychiatry,* 6(3), 214-218.

Tyler, E. B. (1946). Casework with Negro people. *Journal of Social Casework,* 26(7), 265-273.

Vaisbich, S. B. (1978). *Services social, tipologia de diagnostico.* Sao Paulo, Brazil: Cortez & Morales.

Van Der Veen, F. (1967). Basic elements in the process of psychotherapy: A research study. *Journal of Consulting Psychology,* 31(3), 295-303.

Van Fleet, R. (1994). *Filial therapy: Strengthening parent-child relationships through play.* Sarasota, FL: Professional Resource Press.

Varley, B. (1968). The use of role theory in the treatment of disturbed adolescents. *Social Casework,* 49(6), 362-366.

Vasey, I. T. (1968). Developing a data storage and retrieval system. *Social Case-work,* 49(7), 414-417.

Velasquez, R. J., Callahan, W. J., Evans, D., and Ishikuma, T. (1994). DSM-III-R training in master's-level counselling programs. *Psychological Reports,* 74(3), 1331-1338.

Vesper, S. and Spearmann, F. (1966). Treatment of marital conflict resulting from severe personality disturbance. *Social Casework,* 47(9), 583-589.

Vigilante, F. and Mailick, M. (1988). Needs-resource evaluation in the assessment process. *Social Work,* 33(2), 101-104.

Vogel, E. and Bell, N. (1967). The emotionally disturbed child as the family scape-goat. In G. Handel (Ed.), *The psychosocial interior of the family* (pp. 424-440). Chicago: Aldine Publishing Co.

Wachtel, E. (1994). *Treating troubled children and their families.* New York: Guilford Press.

Waldo, M., Brotherton, W. D., and Horswell, R. (1993). Integrating DSM-III-R training into school, marriage and family, and mental health counselor prepara-tion. *Counselor Education and Supervision,* 32, 332-342.

Wasser, E. (1966). Family casework focus on the older person. *Social Casework,* 47(7), 423-431.

Waugh, M. (1967). Psychoanalytic thought on phobia: its evolution and its rele-vance for therapy. *American Journal of Psychiatry,* 123(9), 1075-1080.

Weinberger, J. L. (1958). Basic concepts in diagnosis and treatment of borderline states. In H. J. Parad (Ed.), *Ego psychology and dynamic casework* (pp. 111-116). New York: Family Service Association of America.

Wessel, M. (1963). The unmarried mother: A social work-medical responsibility. *Social Work,* 8(1), 67-71.

West, B. and Rafferty, F. (1958). Initiating therapy with adolescents. *American Journal of Orthopsychiatry,* 28(3), July, 627-639.

Westman, J. C., Kansky, E.W., Erikson, M. E., Arthur, B., and Vroom, A. L. (1963). Parallel group psychotherapy with the parents of emotionally disturbed children. *International Journal of Group Psychotherapy,* 13(1), 52-60.

White, R. (1959). Motivation reconsidered: The concept of competence. *Psycho-logical Review,* 66(5), 297-333.

Widiger, T. A., Frances, A. J., Pincus, H. A., and Davis, W. W. (1990). DSM-IV lit-erature reviews: Rationale, process, and limitations. *Journal of Psychopathology and Behavioral Assessment,* 12(3), 189-202.

Williams, J. B. W. (1981). DSM-III: A comprehensive approach to diagnosis. *So-cial Work,* 26(2), 101-106.

Wodarski, J. S. and Bagarozzi, D. A. (1979). A review of the empirical status of tra-ditional modes of interpersonal helping: implications for social work practice. *Clinical Social Work Journal,* 7(4), 231-255.

Wolberg, L. (1967). *The technique of psychotherapy* (Second edition). New York: Grune and Stratton.

Wolpe, J. (1958). *Psychotherapy by reciprocal inhibition.* Stanford, CA: Stanford University Press.

Wood, K. M. (1971). The contribution of psychoanalysis and ego psychology to social casework. In H. S. Strean (Ed.), *Social casework: Theories in action* (pp. 45-122). Metuchen, NJ: Scarecrow Press.

Woods, M. (1999). *Casework: A psychosocial therapy* (Fifth edition). New York: McGraw-Hill.

Woods, M. and Hollis, F. (1990). *Casework: A psychosocial therapy* (Fourth edition). New York: McGraw-Hill.

Wylie, D. C. and Weinreb, J. (1958). The treatment of a runaway adolescent girl through the treatment of the mother. *American Journal of Orthopsychiatry,* 28(1), January 188-195.

Wylie, M. S. (1995). Diagnosing for dollars? *The Networker,* May-June, 23-27.

Young, L. (1954). *Out of wedlock.* New York: McGraw-Hill.

Zastrow, C. H. (1999). *The practice of social work,* Sixth edition. New York: Brooks/Cole.

Zuckerman, E. L. (1993). *The clinician's thesarus 3.* Pittsburgh, PA: The Clinician's Toolbox.

# Index

# HAWORTH Social Work Practice in Action
Carlton E. Munson, PhD, Senior Editor

**DIAGNOSIS IN SOCIAL WORK: NEW IMPERATIVES** by Francis J. Turner. (2002). "This book is a useful resource for scholars and clinicians involved in clinical social work. It is thoughtfully written and well researched, and a timely additional to the professional literature." *Kathleen J. Farkas, PhD, Associate Professor, Mandel School of Applied Social Sciences, Case Western Reserve University, Cleveland, OH*

**HUMAN BEHAVIOR IN THE SOCIAL ENVIRONMENT: INTERWEAVING THE INNER AND OUTER WORLD** by Esther Urdang. (2002). "This book will serve as a superb introduction to human behavior, normal and pathologic, not only for graduate social work students, but also for anyone who is curious about the vicissitudes of the human condition....The students who use this book will be lucky, indeed." *Calvin A. Colarusso, MD, Clinical Professor of Psychiatry, University of California at San Diego*

**THE USE OF PERSONAL NARRATIVES IN THE HELPING PROFESSIONS: A TEACHING CASEBOOK** by Jessica Heriot and Eileen J. Polinger. (2002). "More than anything else, social work students need examples to connect theories with everyday practice. Here's a book that provides those examples. This book is not only valuable for teaching, it's also an absorbing and instructional pleasure to read." *Leon Ginsberg, PhD, Carolina Distinguished Professor, University of Maryland School of Social Work, Baltimore*

**CHILDREN'S RIGHTS: POLICY AND PRACTICE** by John T. Pardeck. (2001) "Courageous and timely . . . a must-read for everyone concerned not only about the rights of America's children but also about their fate." *Howard Jacob Kerger, PhD, Professor and PhD Director, University of Houston Graduate School of Social Work, Texas*

**BUILDING ON WOMEN'S STRENGTHS: A SOCIAL WORK AGENDA FOR THE TWENTY-FIRST CENTURY, SECOND EDITION** by K. Jean Peterson and Alice A. Lieberman. (2001). "An indispensable resource for courses in women's issues, social work practice with women, and practice from a strengths perspective." *Theresa J. Early, PhD, MSW, Assistant Professor, College of Social Work, Ohio State University, Columbus*

**ELEMENTS OF THE HELPING PROCESS: A GUIDE FOR CLINICIANS, SECOND EDITION** by Raymond Fox. (2001). "Engages the reader with a professional yet easily accessible style. A remarkably fresh, eminently usable set of practical strategies." *Elayne B. Haynes, PhD, ACSW, Assistant Professor, Department of Social Work, Southern Connecticut State University, New Haven*

**SOCIAL WORK THEORY AND PRACTICE WITH THE TERMINALLY ILL, SECOND EDITION** by Joan K. Parry. (2000). "Timely . . . a sensitive and practical approach to working with people with terminal illness and their family members." *Jeanne A.Gill, PhD, LCSW, Adjunct Faculty, San Diego State University, California, and Vice President Southern California Chapter, AASWG*

**WOMEN SURVIVORS, PSYCHOLOGICAL TRAUMA, AND THE POLITICS OF RESISTANCE** by Norma Jean Profitt. (2000). "A compelling argument on the importance of political and collective action as a means of resisting oppression. Should be read by survivors, service providers, and activists in the violence-against-women movement." *Gloria Geller, PhD, Faculty of Social Work, University of Regina, Saskatchewan, Canada*

**THE MENTAL HEALTH DIAGNOSTIC DESK REFERENCE: VISUAL GUIDES AND MORE FOR LEARNING TO USE THE DIAGNOSTIC AND STATISTICAL MANUAL (DSM-IV)** by Carlton E. Munson. (2000). "A carefully organized and user-friendly book for the beginning student and less-experienced practitioner of social work, clinical psychology, of psychiatric nursing . . . It will be a valuable addition to the literature on clinical assessment of mental disorders." *Jerold R. Brandell, PhD, BCD, Professor, School of Social Work, Wayne State University, Detroit, Michigan and Founding Editor, Psychoanalytic Social Work*

**HUMAN SERVICES AND THE AFROCENTRIC PARADIGM** by Jerome H. Schiele. (2000). "Represents a milestone in applying the Afrocentric paradigm to human services generally, and social work specifically. . . . A highly valuable resource." *Bogart R. Leashore, PhD, Dean and Professor, Hunter College School of Social Work, New York, New York*

**SOCIAL WORK: SEEKING RELEVANCY IN THE TWENTY-FIRST CENTURY** by Roland Meinert, John T. Pardeck and Larry Kreuger. (2000). "Highly recommended. A thought-provoking work that asks the difficult questions and challenges the status quo. A great book for graduate students as well as experienced social workers and educators." *Francis K. O. Yuen, DSW, ACSE, Associate Professor, Division of Social Work, California State University, Sacramento*

**SOCIAL WORK PRACTICE IN HOME HEALTH CARE** by Ruth Ann Goode. (2000). "Dr. Goode presents both a lucid scenario and a formulated protocol to bring health care services into the home setting. . . . this is a must have volume that will be a reference to be consulted many times." *Marcia B. Steinhauer, PhD, Coordinator and Associate Professor, Human Services Administration Program, Rider University, Lawrenceville, New Jersey*

**FORSENIC SOCIAL WORK: LEGAL ASPECTS OF PROFESSIONAL PRACTICE, SECOND EDITION** by Robert L. Barker and Douglas M. Branson. (2000). "The authors combine their expertise to create this informative guide to address legal practice issues facing social workers." *Newsletter of the National Organization of Forensic Social Work*

**SOCIAL WORK IN THE HEALTH FIELD: A CARE PERSPECTIVE** by Lois A. Fort Cowles. (1999). "Makes an important contritution to the field by locating the practice of social work in health care within an organizational and social context." *Goldie Kadushin, PhD, Associate Professor, School of Social Welfare, University of Wisconsin, Milwaukee*

**SMART BUT STUCK: WHAT EVERY THERAPY NEEDS TO KNOW ABOUT LEARNING DISABILITIES AND IMPRISONED INTELLIGENCE** by Myrna Orenstein. (1999). "A trailblazing effort that creates an entirely novel way of talking and thinking about learning disabilities. There is simply nothing like it in the field." *Fred M. Levin, MD, Training Supervising Analyst, Chicago Institute for Psychoanalysis; Assistant Professor of Clinical Psychiatry, Northwestern University, School of Medicine, Chicago, IL*

**CLINICAL WORK AND SOCIAL ACTION: AN INTEGRATIVE APPROACH** by Jerome Sachs and Fred Newdom. (1999). "Just in time for the new millennium come Sachs and Newdom with a wholly fresh look at social work. . . . A much-needed uniting of social work values, theories, and practice for action." *Josephine Nieves, MSW, PhD, Executive Director, National Association of Social Workers*

**SOCIAL WORK PRACTICE IN THE MILITARY** by James G. Daley. (1999). "A significant and worthwhile book with provocative and stimulating ideas. It deserves to be read by a wide audience in social work education and practice as well as by decision makers in the military." *H. Wayne Johnson, MSW, Professor, University of Iowa, School of Social Work, Iowa City, Iowa*

**GROUP WORK: SKILLS AND STRATEGIES FOR EFFECTIVE INTERVENTIONS, SECOND EDITION** by Sondra Brandler and Camille P. Roman. (1999). "A clear, basic description of what group work requires, including what skills and techniques group workers need to be effective." *Hospital and Community Psychiatry (from the first edition)*

**TEENAGE RUNAWAYS: BROKEN HEARTS AND "BAD ATTITUDES"** by Laurie Schaffner. (1999). "Skillfully combines the authentic voice of the juvenile runaway with the principles of social science research." *Barbara Owen, PhD, Professor, Department of Criminology, California State University, Fresno*

**CELEBRATING DIVERSITY: COEXISTING IN A MULTICULTURAL SOCIETY** by Benyamin Chetkow-Yanoov. (1999). "Makes a valuable contribution to peace theory and practice." *Ian Harris, EdD, Executive Secretary, Peace Education Committee, International Peace Research Association*

**SOCIAL WELFARE POLICY ANALYSIS AND CHOICES** by Hobart A. Burch. (1999). "Will become the landmark text in its field for many decades to come." *Sheldon Rahan, DSW, Founding Dean and Emeritus Professor of Social Policy and Social Administration, Faculty of Social Work, Wilfrid Laurier University, Canada*

**SOCIAL WORK PRACTICE: A SYSTEMS APPROACH, SECOND EDITION** by Benyamin Chetkow-Yannov. (1999). "Highly recommended as a primary text for any and all introductory social work courses." *Ram A. Cnaan, PhD, Associate Professor, School of Social Work, University of Pennsylvania*

**CRITICAL SOCIAL WELFARE ISSUES: TOOLS FOR SOCIAL WORK AND HEALTH CARE PROFESSIONALS** edited by Arthur J. Katz, Abraham Lurie, and Carlos M. Vida. (1997). "Offers hopeful agendas for change, while navigating the societal challenges facing those in the human services today." *Book News Inc.*

**SOCIAL WORK IN HEALTH SETTINGS: PRACTICE IN CONTEXT, SECOND EDITION** edited by Tobra Schwaber Kerson. (1997). "A first-class document . . . It will be found among the steadier and lasting works on the social work aspects of American health care." *Hans S. Falck, PhD, Professor Emeritus and Former Chair, Health Specialization in Social Work, Virginia Commonwealth University*

**PRINCIPLES OF SOCIAL WORK PRACTICE: A GENERIC PRACTICE APPROACH** by Molly R. Hancock. (1997). "Hancock's discussions advocate reflection and self-awareness to create a climate for client change." *Journal of Social Work Education*

**NOBODY'S CHILDREN: ORPHANS OF THE HIV EPIDEMIC** by Steven F. Dansky. (1997). "Professional sound, moving, and useful for both professionals and interested readers alike." *Ellen G. Friedman, ACSW, Associate Director of Support Services, Beth Israel Medical Center, Methadone Maintenance Treatment Program*

**SOCIAL WORK APPROACHES TO CONFLICT RESOLUTION: MAKING FIGHTING OBSOLETE** by Benyamin Chetkow-yanoov. (1996). "Presents an examination of the nature and cause of conflict and suggests techniques for coping with conflict." *Journal of Criminal Justice*

**FEMINIST THEORIES AND SOCIAL WORK: APPROACHES AND APPLICATIONS** by Christine Flynn Salunier. (1996). "An essential reference to be read repeatedly by all educators and practitioners who are eager to learn more about feminist theory and practice" *Nancy R. Hooyman, PhD, Dean and Professor, School of Social Work, University of Washington, Seattle*

**THE RELATIONAL SYSTEMS MODEL FOR FAMILY THERAPY: LIVING IN THE FOUR REALITIES** by Donald R. Bardill. (1996). "Engages the reader in quiet, thoughtful conversation on the timeless issue of helping families and individuals." *Christian Counseling Resource Review*

**SOCIAL WORK INTERVENTION IN AN ECONOMIC CRISIS: THE RIVER COMMUNITIES PROJECT** by Martha Baum and Pamela Twiss. (1996). "Sets a standard for universities in terms of the types of meaningful roles they can play in supporting and sustaining communities." *Kenneth J. Jaros, PhD, Director, Public Health Social Work Training Program, University of Pittsburgh*

**FUNDAMENTALS OF COGNITIVE-BEHAVIOR THERAPY: FROM BOTH SIDES OF THE DESK** by Bill Borcherdt. (1996). "Both beginning and experienced practitioners . . . will find a considerable number of valuable suggestions in Borcherdt's book." *Albert Ellis, PhD, President, Institute for Rational-Emotive Therapy, New York City*

**BASIC SOCIAL POLICY AND PLANNING: STRATEGIES AND PRACTICE METHODS** by Hobart A. Burch. (1996). "Burch's familiarity with his topic is evident and his book is an easy introduction to the field." *Readings*

**THE CROSS-CULTURAL PRACTICE OF CLINICAL CASE MANAGEMENT IN MENTAL HEALTH** edited by Peter Manoleas. (1996). "Makes a contribution by bringing together the cross-cultural and clinical case management perspectives in working with those who have serious mental illness." *Disabilities Studies Quarterly*

**FAMILY BEYOND FAMILY: THE SURROGATE PARENT IN SCHOOLS AND OTHER COMMUNITY AGENCIES** by Sanford Weinstein. (1995). "Highly recomended to anyone concerned about the welfare of our children and the breakdown of the American family." *Jerold S. Greenberg, EdD, director of Community Service, College of Health & Human Performance, University of Maryland*

**PEOPLE WITH HIV AND THOSE WHO HELP THEM: CHALLENGES, INTEGRATION, INTERVENTION** by R. Dennis Shelby. (1995). "A useful and compassionate contribution to the HIV psychotherapy literature." *Public Health*

**THE BLACK ELDERLY: SATISFACTION AND QUALITY OF LATER LIFE** by Marguerite Coke and James A. Twaite. (1995). "Presents a model for predicting life satisfaction in this population." *Abstracts in Social Gerontology*

**NOW DARE EVERYTHING: TALES OF HIV-RELATED PSYCHOTHER-APY** by Steven F. Dansky. (1994). "A highly recommended book for anyone working with persons who are HIV positive. . . . Every library should have a copy of this book." *AIDS Book Review Journal*

**INTERVENTION RESEARCH: DESIGN AND DEVELOPMENT FOR HU-MAN SERVICE** edited by Jack Rothman and Edwin J. Thomas. (1994). "Provides a useful framework for the further examination of methodology for each separate step of such research." *Academic Library Book Review*

**CLINICAL SOCIAL WORK SUPERVISION, SECOND EDITION** by Carlton E. Munson. (1993). "A useful, thorough, and articulate reference for supervisors and for 'supervisees' who are wanting to understand their supervisor or are looking for effective supervision...." *Transactional Analysis Journal*

**IF A PARTNER HAS AIDS: GUIDE TO CLINICAL INTERVENTION FOR RELATIONSHIPS IN CRISIS** by R. Dennis Shelby. (1993). "A women addition to existing publications about couples coping with AIDS, it offers intervention ideas and strategies to clinicians." *Contemporary Psychology*

**GERONTOLOGICAL SOCIAL WORK SUPERVISION** by Ann Burack-Weiss and Frances Coyle Brennan. (1991). "The creative ideas in this book will aid supervisiors working with students and experienced social workers." *Senior News*

**THE CREATIVE PRACTITIONER: THEORY AND METHODS FOR THE HELPING SERVICES** by Bernard Gelfand. (1988). "[Should] be widely adopted by those in the helping services. It could lead to significant positive advances by countless individuals." *Sidney J. Parnes, Trustee Chairperson for Strategic Program Development, Creative Education Foundation, Buffalo, NY*

**MANAGEMENT AND INFORMATION SYSTEMS IN HUMAN SERVICES: IMPLICATIONS FOR THE DISTRIBUTION OF AUTHORITY AND DECISION MAKING** by Richard K. Caputo. (1987). "A contribution to social work scholarship in that it provides conceptual frameworks that can be used in the design of management information systems." *Social Work*

## Order a copy of this book with this form or online at:
http://www.haworthpressinc.com/store/product.asp?sku=4539

# DIAGNOSIS IN SOCIAL WORK
## New Imperatives

_____in hardbound at $39.95 (ISBN: 0-7890-0871-8)

_____in softbound at $24.95 (ISBN: 0-7890-1596-X)

COST OF BOOKS_____

OUTSIDE USA/CANADA/
MEXICO: ADD 20%____

POSTAGE & HANDLING_____
*(US: $4.00 for first book & $1.50
for each additional book)
Outside US: $5.00 for first book
& $2.00 for each additional book)*

SUBTOTAL_____

in Canada: add 7% GST____

STATE TAX____
*(NY, OH & MIN residents, please
add appropriate local sales tax)*

**FINAL TOTAL____**
*(If paying in Canadian funds,
convert using the current
exchange rate, UNESCO
coupons welcome.)*

**BILL ME LATER:** ($5 service charge will be added)
(Bill-me option is good on US/Canada/Mexico orders only;
not good to jobbers, wholesalers, or subscription agencies.)

Check here if billing address is different from
shipping address and attach purchase order and
billing address information.

Signature_____

**PAYMENT ENCLOSED: $_____**

**PLEASE CHARGE TO MY CREDIT CARD.**

Visa        MasterCard        AmEx        Discover
            Diner's Club        Eurocard        JCB

Account # _____

Exp. Date_____

Signature_____

Prices in US dollars and subject to change without notice.

NAME_____

INSTITUTION_____

ADDRESS_____

CITY_____

STATE/ZIP_____

COUNTRY_____ COUNTY (NY residents only)_____

TEL_____ FAX_____

E-MAIL_____

May we use your e-mail address for confirmations and other types of information?    Yes    No
We appreciate receiving your e-mail address and fax number. Haworth would like to e-mail or fax special
discount offers to you, as a preferred customer. **We will never share, rent, or exchange your e-mail address
or fax number.** We regard such actions as an invasion of your privacy.

*Order From Your Local Bookstore or Directly From*
**The Haworth Press, Inc.**
10 Alice Street, Binghamton, New York 13904-1580 • USA
TELEPHONE: 1-800-HAWORTH (1-800-429-6784) / Outside US/Canada: (607) 722-5857
FAX: 1-800-895-0582 / Outside US/Canada: (607) 722-6362
E-mail: getinfo@haworthpressinc.com
PLEASE PHOTOCOPY THIS FORM FOR YOUR PERSONAL USE.
www.HaworthPress.com

BOF00